The Diabetes Dictionary

What Every Person
with Diabetes
Needs to Know

AMERICAN
DIABETES
ASSOCIATION

Writer, Gregory L. Guthrie; *Managing Editor, Book Publishing*, Abe Ogden; *Acquisitions Editor, Consumer Books*, Robert Anthony; *Production Manager*, Melissa Sprott; *Composition*, ADA; *Cover Design*, ADA; *Printer*, Worzalla Publishing.

Printed in the United States of America
1 3 5 7 9 10 8 6 4 2

The suggestions and information contained in this publication are generally consistent with the Clinical Practice Recommendations and other policies of the American Diabetes Association, but they do not represent the policy or position of the Association or any of its boards or committees. Reasonable steps have been taken to ensure the accuracy of the information presented. However, the American Diabetes Association cannot ensure the safety or efficacy of any product or service described in this publication. Individuals are advised to consult a physician or other appropriate health care professional before undertaking any diet or exercise program or taking any medication referred to in this publication. Professionals must use and apply their own professional judgment, experience, and training and should not rely solely on the information contained in this publication before prescribing any diet, exercise, or medication. The American Diabetes Association—its officers, directors, employees, volunteers, and members—assumes no responsibility or liability for personal or other injury, loss, or damage that may result from the suggestions or information in this publication.

⊛ The paper in this publication meets the requirements of the ANSI Standard Z39.48-1992 (permanence of paper).

ADA titles may be purchased for business or promotional use or for special sales. To purchase more than 50 copies of this book at a discount, or for custom editions of this book with your logo, contact Lee Romano Sequeira, Special Sales & Promotions, at the address below, by e-mail at LRomano@diabetes.org, or by calling 703-299-2046.

For all other inquiries, please call 1-800-DIABETES.

American Diabetes Association
1701 North Beauregard Street
Alexandria, Virginia 22311

Library of Congress Cataloging-in-Publication Data

The diabetes dictionary / American Diabetes Association.
    p. cm.
  Includes bibliographical references and index.
  ISBN 978-1-58040-252-1 (alk. paper)
  1. Diabetes—Dictionaries. I. American Diabetes Association.

RC660.D445 2007
616.4'62003—dc22

2007011918

CONTENTS

Why We Wrote This Book
v

How to Use This Book
vii

The Diabetes Dictionary
1

List of Common
Acronyms and Abbreviations
142

WHY WE
WROTE THIS BOOK

Dealing with the day-to-day worries and burdens of diabetes is often enough to overwhelm the hardiest of souls. It's tough enough conquering the initial feelings that arise with a diagnosis of diabetes and listening to those subtle symptoms and signs that your body is telling you. How do I take care of myself? Is my blood sugar low? Is it high? That's a lot to take on. On top of all of that, it often seems like the people who are experts in diabetes and who care for people with diabetes know and speak a totally different language.

In a lot of ways, thinking about diabetes will at first seem like visiting a foreign country. Everyone speaks a different language and operates under an unfamiliar set of rules. Yet, when you get a grip on the native language and the customs, you begin to understand why people do the things they do. It suddenly begins to make sense.

That's why we wrote this book. We want you to understand the native language that surrounds the world of diabetes.

When you read a newspaper story, find a story in a magazine, watch a report on the evening news, or come across an article on the Internet on diabetes, you're likely to see and hear a great deal of words, terms, and phrases that you may not understand. If you're looking at recent scientific research in diabetes, you'll find even more obscure and strange words. It's likely that you will encounter many words that you've never even seen or heard before. With this book, we've set out to give you common-sense, straightforward definitions for many of the words that are common in discussions about diabetes.

The goal of the American Diabetes Association is to provide you with the tools you need to make proper diabetes self-care an achievable reality in the foreseeable future. Knowledge is one of those tools, and with this dictionary, you will begin to understand what diabetes is, how it works, why it happens, and how to take care of it.

HOW TO USE THIS BOOK

GENERAL TIPS

This dictionary has been put together much like any of the other dictionaries you may have used over the course of your life. The entries are sorted alphabetically. The shaded tabs along the outer margin of the pages indicate the letter range that is covered within those pages. This allows for quicker, more precise browsing.

Terms that are represented numerically are listed under the letter that begins the first number. Therefore, in the case of *504 Plan*, this entry is listed under "five" in the "F" section.

In many cases, you will find that diabetes-specific terms that are used in the definitions will themselves be defined elsewhere in the book. So, for example, the definition for *alpha-tocopherol* uses the term *antioxidant*, which has its own entry in this dictionary.

GUIDE WORDS

At the top of each page of entries, you will find the familiar guide words that are common to all dictionaries. On the left-hand page, the guide word will identify the first word that has a definition beginning on that page. On the right-hand page, the guide word will identify the last word that has a definition beginning on that page. Using these will allow you to quickly locate your desired entry.

LIST OF COMMON ACRONYMS AND ABBREVIATIONS

Many of the terms common in discussions about diabetes are referred to in their acronym forms or as abbreviations. An acronym is created by combining successively the first letters of a series of words (e.g., ARB is an acronym for *angiotensin receptor blocker*). In most cases, the acronym or abbreviation is referenced only in the entry for the full term, so you will not find it as an individual entry (e.g., there is no individual entry for ARB). To aid you in finding the definition for terms that are often referred to as acronyms, a list of common acronyms and abbreviations is included at the end of the book. Simply find the acronym or abbreviation for which you are looking, read across to see the full term, and find the entry for the full term.

PRONUNCIATION

After the entry name, a phonetic pronunciation guide has been provided in parentheses. The pronunciation guides are meant to be easy to read and to understand, so they may not precisely correlate with those found in other dictionaries. In general, individual elements separated by hyphens (-) indicate an individual syllable, but this is not always true. Elements present in all capital (or uppercase) letters represent an element that is said with emphasis. Typically, when attempting to pronounce an entry using the pronunciation guide, just try to speak each element aloud as written.

ABBREVIATIONS USED IN THIS BOOK

In many cases, abbreviations are used within individual entries to identify common pieces of information that broaden the understanding of a term, such as an example, a synonym, or a common abbreviation. The following is a list of the abbreviations used in the entries of this dictionary.

ABBREV.:	abbreviation or acronym
B.N.:	brand or trade name (of a drug)
e.g.:	"for example"
Ex.:	examples include
G.N.:	generic name (of a drug)
ANT.:	antonym; a word with nearly the opposite meaning
OBS.:	uncommon or obsolete; a word that is no longer in common use
SYN.:	synonym; a word with nearly the same meaning

A

A1C test (AY-wan-see tehst): a test that shows a person's average blood glucose level over the past 2–3 months, usually shown as a percentage. The A1C test measures the amount of glycosylated hemoglobin (also called hemoglobin A1C, glycated hemoglobin, or HbA_{1c}) in the blood.

acanthosis nigricans (uh-kan-THO-sis NIH-grih-kans): a skin condition characterized by darkened skin patches. Common in people whose body is not responding correctly to the insulin that they make in their pancreas (insulin resist-

A–E

ance). This skin condition is also seen in people who have pre-diabetes or type 2 diabetes.

acarbose (AK-er-bose): a drug from the class of oral diabetes medications called alpha-glucosidase inhibitors. Used to treat people with type 2 diabetes by blocking the enzymes that digest starches (carbohydrates) in food. B.N.: Precose.

ACE inhibitor (AY-ss in-hib-it-or): an oral medicine that lowers blood pressure. ACE stands for angiotensin-converting enzyme. For people with diabetes, especially those who have protein (albumin) in the urine, it also helps slow down kidney damage.

acesulfame potassium (AY-see-SUL-fame puh-TAS-ee-um): a low-calorie sweetener with no calories and no nutritional value. B.N.: Sunett. SYN.: acesulfame-K.

acetohexamide (a-see-toh-HEX-uh-myde): an oral diabetes medicine used to treat type 2 diabetes that belongs to the sulfonylurea class of medications. B.N.: Dymelor.

acute (a-CUTE): something that happens suddenly and for a short time; often accompanied by a sharp rise in severity. ANT.: chronic.

Adequate Intake (ad-eh-qwit in-tayke): one of the four reference values for the Dietary Reference Intake based on observed or experimentally determined estimates of nutrient intake by a group of healthy people that are assumed to be adequate; used when a Recommended Dietary Allowance cannot be determined. ABBREV.: AI.

adhesive capsulitis (ad-HEE-sive cap-soo-LITE-iss): a condition of the shoulder associated with diabetes; results in pain and loss of the ability to move the shoulder in all directions.

adipose tissue (ad-uh-POHS tis-SHOO): commonly referred to as fat; a connective tissue that stores fat for energy, insulation, and cushioning.

adult-onset diabetes (ad-ulht-on-set DY-uh-beet-eez): OBS.; SYN.: type 2 diabetes.

advanced glycosylation end product (ad-vans-d gly-KOH-sih-lay-shun end prah-duct): a product created in the body when glucose links with protein; plays a role in damaging blood vessels, which can lead to diabetes complications. ABBREV.: AGE.

aerobic exercise (air-OH-bick ecks-er-size): rapid physical activity that stresses the heart, lungs, arms, legs, and the rest of the body; typically causes harder breathing and faster heart rate. *Ex.*: dancing, jogging, running, swimming, walking, bicycling.

albumin (al-BYOO-min): a protein found in animal tissues, manufactured by the liver and circulated in human blood.

albumin excretion rate (al-BYOO-min ECKS-cree-shun rayte): a urine test that measures the amount of albumin in the urine in order to determine kidney function. ABBREV.: AER.

albuminuria (al-BYOO-mih-NOO-ree-uh): a condition in which the urine has more than normal amounts of albumin; a frequent sign of diabetic nephropathy (kidney disease).

alpha cell (AL-fa sel): a type of cell in the pancreas that makes and releases a hormone called glucagon. The body sends a signal to the alpha cells to make glucagon when blood glucose levels fall too low, then glucagon reaches the liver, which releases glucose into the blood for energy. Also written as α-cell.

alpha-glucosidase inhibitor (AL-fa gloo-KOH-sih-days in-hib-it-or): a class of oral medicine for type 2 diabetes that blocks the enzymes that digest starches in food. The result is a slower and lower rise in blood glucose throughout the day, especially right after meals. G.N.: acarbose, miglitol. Also written as α-glucosidase inhibitor.

alpha-tocopherol (AL-fa toe-co-fir-all): a biologically active form of vitamin E and powerful antioxidant. Also written as α-tocopherol.

alternative medicine (all-turn-eh-tiv med-ih-sin): a branch of complementary and alternative medicine that is used in place of conventional treatments for medical conditions. *Ex.*: following a special diet to treat a disease rather than undergoing surgery.

amino acid (uh-MEAN-oh ass-id): the basic building block of protein; 20 different amino acids are commonly found in proteins.

amputation (am-PEW-tay-shun): the removal by surgery of one or more limbs or of the digits (e.g., fingers and toes).

amylin (AM-ih-lin): a hormone formed by beta cells in the pancreas; regulates the timing of glucose release into the bloodstream after eating by slowing the emptying of the stomach.

amyotrophy (AY-me-uh-treh-fee): a type of neuropathy resulting in pain, weakness, and/or wasting in the muscles.

analog (anna-log): SYN.: insulin analog.

anemia (uh-NEE-mee-uh): a condition in which the number of red blood cells is less than normal, resulting in less oxygen being carried to the body's cells.

angina (an-JI-na): chest pain that arises from reduced blood flow to the heart (ischemia), often due to cardiovascular disease. SYN.: angina pectoris.

angiopathy (an-gee-AH-puh-thee): any disease of the blood vessels (veins, arteries, and capillaries) or lymphatic vessels.

angioplasty (an-gee-UH-plast-EE): surgical procedure to repair a blocked or narrowed blood vessel. During this noninvasive procedure, a balloon-tipped catheter (thin tube) is introduced into the blood vessel. When the balloon inflates, the vessel widens, thus allowing improved blood flow. Also called balloon angioplasty, coronary angioplasty, and percutaneous transluminal coronary angioplasty.

angiotensin (an-gee-oh-TEN-sin): a polypeptide in the blood that constricts the blood vessels and thereby increases blood pressure.

angiotensin-converting enzyme (an-gee-oh-TEN-sin con-VERT-ing EN-zime): SYN.: ACE inhibitor.

angiotensin receptor blocker (an-gee-oh-TEN-sin REE-sep-tur block-er): an oral medicine that is used to treat hypertension. ABBREV.: ARB.

A–E

anorexia nervosa (AN-or-ecks-ee-uh ner-VOSE-uh): an eating disorder in which people refrain from eating in order to stay thin and prevent weight gain; can lead to unpredictable blood glucose levels and diabetes complications.

antibody (AN-tee-bod-ee): a protein made by the body to protect itself from foreign substances, such as bacteria or viruses.

antigen (an-TIH-jen): a foreign substance that, when introduced to the body, elicits the production of antibodies.

antihypertensive drug (AN-tee-HI-per-ten-siv drug): any of a class of medications that lowers blood pressure to treat hypertension, including ACE inhibitors, beta blockers, ARBs, calcium antagonists, calcium channel blockers, and thiazide diuretics.

antioxidant (AN-tee-ox-ih-dent): chemical substance that helps protect against cell damage caused by free radicals. *Ex.*: vitamin A, vitamin C, and vitamin E.

apoptosis (ap-OH-toe-sis): a normal cell process that involves a genetically programmed series of events that lead to the death of a cell, sometimes called cell suicide.

arteriosclerosis (ar-TEER-ee-oh-skluh-RO-sis): hardening of the arteries.

artery (ar-ter-ee): a large blood vessel that carries blood with oxygen from the heart to all parts of the body.

aspart insulin (ASS-part IN-suh-lin): a rapid-acting insulin that, on average, starts to lower blood glucose levels within 10–20 minutes after injection, has its strongest effect 30–60 minutes after injection, and keeps working for 3–5 hours after injection. B.N.: Novolog.

aspartame (ASS-per-tame): a low-calorie sweetener with almost no calories and almost no nutritional value. B.N.: Equal, NutraSweet.

aspirin therapy (ASS-per-in thair-uh-pee): a form of preventive treatment in which a low dose of aspirin (75–162 mg) is prescribed daily to reduce the risks of heart attacks, which is a frequent complication in people with diabetes.

atherectomy (ATH-eh-wreck-TOW-me): a nonsurgical procedure in which a rotating blade is used to remove plaque from the walls of hardened or clogged arteries; used to treat atherosclerosis.

atherosclerosis (ATH-eh-row-skleh-RO-sis): clogging, narrowing, and hardening of the body's large arteries and medium-sized blood vessels; can lead to coronary artery disease, resulting in stroke, heart attack, eye problems, and kidney problems.

atypical antipsychotic agents (AY-tip-ih-cull an-TI-sigh-cot-ic AY-jents): a class of drug used to treat schizophrenia and other psychoses that has been associated with increased risk of developing type 2 diabetes.

autoantibody (AW-tow-AN-tee-bod-ee): a self-recognizing antibody that targets and attacks the cells of the body, leading the body to attack itself; three autoantibodies are particularly common in those with type 1 diabetes: islet cell autoantibodies, insulin autoantibodies, and glutamic acid decarboxylase.

autoimmune disease (AW-tow-ih-MYOON dih-zeez): disorder in which the body's immune system mistakenly attacks and destroys body tissue that it believes to be foreign.

autonomic neuropathy (aw-tow-NOM-ik ne-ROP-uh-thee): a form of neuropathy that affects the lungs, heart, stomach, intestines, bladder, or genitals.

B

background insulin (bak-grownd IN-suh-lin): SYN.: basal insulin.

background retinopathy (bak-grownd REH-tih-NOP-uh-thee): a type of damage to the retina of the eye marked by bleeding, fluid accumulation, and abnormal dilation of the blood vessels; often results in blurred vision; an early stage of diabetic retinopathy; also called simple or nonproliferative retinopathy.

bacteria (back-TEER-ee-uh): very small, single-celled life-forms that can reproduce quickly and can cause some diseases. Also called germs.

balloon angioplasty (ba-LOON an-gee-OH-plast-EE): SYN.: angioplasty.

bariatrics (BARE-ee-at-ricks) the branch of medicine that deals with the causes, prevention, and treatment of obesity.

basal insulin (BAY-suhl IN-suh-lin): **1.** an intermediate- or long-acting insulin that is absorbed slowly and gives the body a steady, low level of insulin to manage blood glucose levels between meals, thus mimicking the body's natural low-level steady background release of insulin; background insulin. **2.** the low-level steady background release of insulin by an insulin pump.

basal rate (BAY-suhl rayte): a steady trickle of low levels of rapid-acting insulin, such as that used in an insulin pump.

B cell (BEE sel): a lymphocyte that produces antibodies; sometimes it mistakenly creates autoantibodies, which may be involved in the development of diabetes. SYN.: B lymphocyte.

behavioral therapy (BEE-hayve-your-ul thair-uh-pee): an approach to treatment in which specific behaviors are targeted for change, including the ideas and emotions associated with that behavior; often used to adjust eating habits in order to encourage weight loss.

beta blocker (BAY-tuh block-er): an antihypertensive drug.

beta cell (BAY-tuh sel): a cell that makes insulin and amylin and is located in the islet cells of the pancreas. Also written as β-cell.

biguanide (by-GWAH-nide): a class of oral medicine used to treat type 2 diabetes that lowers blood glucose by reducing the amount of glucose produced by the liver and by helping the body respond better to insulin. G.N.: metformin.

blood fat (blud fat): a lipid carried through the blood by a lipoprotein; usually used to refer to cholesterol and triglyceride.

blood glucose (blud GLOO-kose): the main sugar found in the blood and the body's main energy source; also called blood sugar. ABBREV.: BG.

blood glucose level (blud GLOO-kose lev-el): the amount of glucose in a given amount of blood; often measured in milligrams of glucose per deciliter of blood and shown as mg/dl.

blood glucose meter (blud GLOO-kose mee-tur): a small, portable machine used by people with diabetes to frequently check their blood glucose levels. After pricking the skin with a lancet, one places a drop of blood on a test strip in the machine, and then the meter (or monitor) soon displays the blood glucose level on a digital display. SYN.: glucometer.

blood glucose monitoring (blud GLOO-kose mon-ih-ter-ing): the process and procedure of frequently and regularly checking blood glucose levels in order to manage diabetes, usually with the aid of a blood glucose meter or blood glucose test strips that change color when touched by a blood sample.

blood pressure (blud preh-shure): the force of blood exerted on the inside walls of blood vessels. It is expressed as a ratio (e.g., 120/80 mmHg, read as "120 over 80") in millimeters of mercury. The first number is the systolic (sis-TAH-lik) pressure—the pressure when the heart pushes blood out into the arteries—and the second number is the diastolic (DY-uh-STAH-lik) pressure—the pressure when the heart rests. ABBREV.: BP.

blood sugar (blud shoog-ur): SYN.: blood glucose.

blood urea nitrogen (blud yoo-REE-uh NY-truh-jen): a waste product in the blood that results from the breakdown of protein (urea); normally filtered out of the blood by the kidneys and eliminated from the body in the urine. Blood urea nitrogen levels are measured to evaluated kidney function; increasing levels indicate decreasing kidney function. ABBREV.: BUN.

blood vessel (blud vess-el): any of the many tubes that carry blood to and from all parts of the body, including arteries, veins, and capillaries.

body mass index (bah-dee mass in-dex): a method of evaluating the body's weight relative to its height and represented as weight in kilograms divided by the square of the height in meters (kg/m^2); used to determine the following categories: underweight, normal weight, overweight, or obese. This measurement correlates highly with body fat. ABBREV.: BMI.

bolus insulin (BOH-lus IN-suh-lin): an extra amount of insulin taken to cover an expected rise in blood glucose, often related to a meal or snack.

borderline diabetes (bore-dur-line DY-uh-beet-eez): OBS.; SYN.: type 2 diabetes, impaired glucose tolerance, or impaired fasting glucose.

brittle diabetes (brit-ull DY-uh-beet-eez): a condition in people with diabetes wherein blood glucose levels swing wildly and unpredictably high or low; the advent of blood glucose monitoring has made this condition uncommon. SYN.: labile or unstable diabetes.

bulimia (buh-leem-ee-uh): an eating disorder distinguished by binging behavior (consuming large amounts of food) and then purging behavior, including vomiting, laxative use, and/or excessive exercise; can lead to unpredictable blood glucose levels and diabetes complications.

bunion (BUN-yun): a bulge on the first joint of the big toe, caused by the swelling of a fluid sac under the skin and due to genetically weakened joints or ill-fitting shoes; such a spot can become red, sore, and infected; can lead to serious foot infections if left untreated.

C

C-peptide (see pep-tide): Abbreviation for "connecting peptide," a substance released by the beta cells into the bloodstream in amounts equal to that of insulin; testing levels of C-peptide reveals how much insulin the body is making.

C-reactive protein (see ree-act-iv PRO-teen): a protein found in the blood that is a marker for inflammation; its presence indicates a heightened state of inflammation in the body. ABBREV.: CRP.

calcium (kal-SEE-um): mineral that gives strength to bones and teeth and has an important role in muscle contraction, blood clotting, and nerve function.

calcium antagonist (kal-SEE-um an-TAG-un-ist): a class of antihypertensive drug.

calcium channel blocker (kal-SEE-um chan-uhl-block-er): a class of antihypertensive drug.

callus (CAL-us): a small area of skin, usually on the foot, that has become thick and hard from rubbing or pressure.

calorie (CAL-or-ee): a unit of measurement for the energy provided by food; carbohydrate, protein, fat, and alcohol provide calories to the diet. Carbohydrate and protein have 4 calories per gram, fat has 9 calories per gram, and alcohol has 7 calories per gram. SYN.: kilocalorie.

capillary (KAP-ih-lair-ee): the smallest of the blood vessels. Oxygen and glucose pass through capillary walls and enter the body's cells, and waste products, such as carbon dioxide, exit the cells through capillary walls and enter the blood.

capillary blood glucose monitoring (KAP-ih-lair-ee blud GLOO-kose mon-ih-ter-ing): a method of blood glucose monitoring that is usually conducted in hospitalized patients by nurses and other practitioners. ABBREV.: CBGM.

capsaicin (kap-SAY-ih-sin): an ingredient in hot peppers that can be found in ointment form for use on the skin to relieve pain from diabetic neuropathy.

carbohydrate (kar-bow-HY-drate): one of the three primary nutrients found in food, primarily starches, vegetables, fruits, dairy products, and sugars. ABBREV.: CHO, carb.

carbohydrate counting (kar-bow-HY-drate cown-ting): method of meal planning for people with diabetes based on counting the number of grams of carbohydrate in the food that is consumed.

carbohydrate-to-insulin ratio (kar-bow-HY-drate-too-IN-suh-lin ray-she-oh): a ratio used to determine how many units of bolus insulin a person with diabetes needs to take in order to

A–E

cover the effect of 10 grams of carbohydrate on blood glucose levels.

cardiologist (kar-dee-AH-luh-jist): a doctor who treats people who have heart problems.

cardiometabolic risk factors (KAR-dee-oh-MET-ah-BALL-ick rizk fack-tors): a set of risk factors that, when viewed together, are good indicators of a person's overall risk of developing heart disease and type 2 diabetes. These risk factors include obesity, high LDL cholesterol, high triglycerides, low HDL cholesterol, hypertension, smoking, and physical inactivity. Each of these risk factors poses a danger to good health, and the more one has, the greater the risk of heart disease and type 2 diabetes.

cardiomyopathy (KAR-dee-oh-my-ah-puh-thee): a heart disease in which the heart is weakened and does not function properly.

cardiovascular disease (KAR-dee-oh-VASK-yoo-ler dih-zeez): disease of the heart and blood vessels (arteries, veins, and capillaries). ABBREV.: CVD.

cataract (KA-ter-act): clouding of the lens of the eye.

celiac disease (see-lee-ak dih-zeez): a condition in which gluten damages the intestines, an organ that helps digest food, and therefore nutrients are not absorbed properly, which leads to many other complications. Celiac disease arises more frequently in people with type 1 diabetes and is generally treated by prescribing a gluten-free diet. SYN.: celiac sprue, nontropical sprue, or gluten-sensitive enteropathy.

cerebral embolism (seh-REE-brul em-bowl-izm): a blood clot from one part of the body that is carried by the bloodstream to the brain where it blocks an artery; can cause a stroke.

cerebrovascular disease (seh-REE-broh-VASK-yoo-ler dih-zeez): damage to blood vessels in the brain that can interrupt blood flow to the brain, which can result in a stroke.

certified diabetes educator (ser-tih-fyed DY-uh-beet-eez ed-joo-kay-tor): a health care professional with expertise in diabetes education and who has met eligibility requirements and successfully completed a certification exam. ABBREV.: CDE.

A–E

Charcot's foot (shar-KOHZ foot): a condition in which the joints and soft tissue in the foot are destroyed; caused by damage to the nerves.

chemical diabetes (kem-ih-cul DY-uh-beet-eez): OBS.; SYN.: impaired glucose tolerance.

chlorpropamide (klor-PROH-pah-mide): an oral medicine used to treat type 2 diabetes that belongs to the class of medicines called sulfonylureas. B.N.: Diabinese.

cholesterol (koh-LES-ter-all): a type of fat produced by the liver and found in the blood; it is also found in foods from animals; used by the body to make hormones and build cell walls.

chronic (KRON-ick): something that is long lasting. Because no known cure exists for diabetes, it is considered a chronic (long-lasting) disease. ANT.: acute.

chronic obstructive pulmonary disease (KRON-ick ub-STRUCK-tive puhl-mun-air-ee dih-zeez): a lung disease in which the airways in the lungs produce excess mucus resulting in frequent coughing; a majority of the risk for developing this disease comes from smoking. ABBREV.: COPD.

circulation (sir-cue-lay-shun): the flow of blood through the body's blood vessels and heart.

co-insurance (KOH-in-shur-ens): a co-payment for fee-for-service health plans, usually represented as a percentage of cost (e.g., the insurance company pays 75% of the claim and the insured pays the remaining 25%) and applied after the plan's deductible has been met.

coma (KOH-mah): a sleep-like state in which a person is not conscious; can be caused by severe hyperglycemia or hypoglycemia in people with diabetes.

combination medicine (kom-bih-nay-shun med-ih-sin): a pill that includes two or more different medicines; often used to reduce costs and the number of pills a patient takes.

combination therapy (kom-bih-nay-shun thair-uh-pee): the use of different medicines together, such as multiple oral hypoglycemic agents or one oral hypoglycemic agent and insulin, to manage the blood glucose levels in people with type 2 diabetes.

complementary and alternative medicine (kom-plih-men-tair-ee and all-turn-eh-tiv med-ih-sin): a broad group of medical and health care systems, practices, and products that are not presently considered to be part of conventional medicine because of unproven and insufficient research-based evidence. *Ex.*: aromatherapy, yoga, dietary supplements. ABBREV.: CAM.

complication (kom-plih-kay-shun): a harmful, but preventable, condition that results from the effects of diabetes on the body, such as damage to the eyes, heart, blood vessels, nervous system, teeth, gums, feet, skin, and kidneys.

Consolidated Omnibus Budget Reconciliation Act (kun-sahl-ih-day-ted AHM-nee-bus buhd-jet reh-kon-sil-ee-ay-shun ackt): a federal law enacted in 1986. Under this act, an employer with more than 20 employees must allow a former employee and his or her dependents to retain the same health insurance policy with equal coverage for 18–36 months after leaving the job. The former employee has to pay for the coverage and may be charged up to 2%

more than the rate charged to the employer. ABBREV.: COBRA.

congenital defect (kun-JEN-ih-tul dee-fekt): problem or condition that is present at birth.

congestive heart failure (kun-jes-tiv hart FAYL-yur): loss of the heart's pumping power, which causes fluids to collect in the body, especially in the feet and lungs. ABBREV.: CHF.

connecting peptide (kun-eckt-ing pep-tide): SYN.: C-peptide.

continuous glucose monitoring system (kun-tin-YOO-us gloo-KOSE mon-ih-ter-ing SIS-tem): a device that continuously records blood glucose levels throughout the day and night through a subcutaneously implanted sensor. The system is used to measure average blood glucose levels for up to 3 days in order to help identify fluctuations and trends that would otherwise go unnoticed with standard A1C tests and fingerstick measurements. ABBREV.: CGMS.

continuous subcutaneous insulin infusion
(kun-tin-YOO-us sub-kyoo-TAY-nee-us IN-suh-lin in-fyoo-zhun): the method by which insulin
pumps deliver insulin. A steady, measured
amount of basal insulin is delivered under the
skin (subcutaneously). ABBREV.: CSII.

contraindication (KON-tra-in-dih-KAY-shun): a
condition or situation that increases the risks
involved in using a particular drug, carrying
out a medical procedure, or engaging in a particular activity, thus making the treatment
inadvisable.

conventional therapy (kun-ven-shun-uhl thair-uh-
pee): a term used in clinical trials in which one
group receives treatment for diabetes in which
A1C and blood glucose levels are kept at levels based on current practice guidelines. The
goal is not to keep blood glucose levels as close
to normal as possible, as is done in intensive
therapy. Conventional therapy includes use of
medication, meal planning, and exercise, along
with regular visits to health care providers.

co-payment (KOH-pay-ment): a method of shar-
ing costs between an insurance company and

its members; often a discounted flat fee paid every time the member receives a medical service.

corn (kohrn): a callus on the toe.

coronary angioplasty (kohr-uh-nair-ee an-gee-UH-plast-EE): SYN.: angioplasty.

coronary artery (kohr-uh-nair-ee ar-ter-ee): any one of the many blood vessels that brings oxygen-rich blood to the heart to keep it functioning and healthy.

coronary artery bypass graft (kohr-uh-nair-ee ar-ter-ee BYE-pass graft): a surgical procedure in which a healthy blood vessel is transplanted from another part of the body (usually the legs) into the heart to replace or bypass a diseased one. ABBREV.: CABG.

coronary artery disease (kohr-uh-nair-ee ar-ter-ee dih-zeez): condition in which atherosclerosis of the coronary arteries has significantly reduced or restricted blood flow to the heart, thus leading to angina or myocardial infarction. ABBREV.: CAD.

coronary heart disease (kohr-uh-nair-ee hart dih-zeez): condition caused by narrowing of the arteries that supply blood to the heart; can result in a heart attack. ABBREV.: CHD.

corticosteroid (kore-tih-KO-stair-OYD): a steroid produced by the adrenal glands that suppresses inflammation; helps maintain blood glucose levels, blood pressure, and muscle strength; and controls salt and water balance.

cortisol (KORT-ih-sawl): a glucocorticoid; a hormone produced by the adrenal gland; commercially manufactured as hydrocortisone and used to reduce inflammation.

counterregulatory hormone (kown-tur-reg-yool-uh-tore-ee HORE-mowne): a hormone released during stressful situations, including glucagon, epinephrine (adrenaline), norepinephrine, cortisol, and growth hormone. Such hormones tell the liver to release glucose and the fat cells to release fatty acids for extra energy. If the body does not have enough insulin present when these hormones are released, hyperglycemia and diabetic ketoacidosis can result.

Coxsackie virus (KOK-sax-ee VY-rus): any of the family of viruses related to the one that causes polio. The Coxsackie B4 virus has a small region of protein that is almost identical to a region of the glutamic acid decarboxylase molecule and therefore is suspected to have some connection to the autoimmune response in type 1 diabetes.

creatinine (kree-AT-ih-nin): a waste product from protein in the diet and from the muscles of the body that is eliminated from the body by the kidneys in the form of urine; used as a marker for kidney function because as nephropathy progresses, the creatinine levels in the blood increase.

Cushing's syndrome (koosh-ingz sin-drohm): a hormonal disorder caused by excessive exposure of the body's tissues to the hormone cortisol and characterized by accumulation of fat around the abdomen and upper back. This increased body weight can put people at risk of developing type 2 diabetes.

cyclosporine (SY-kloh-SPOR-een): an immunosuppressant drug.

cystic fibrosis (SYS-tick FY-bro-sis): a genetic disorder in which mucus in the body becomes thick, dry, and sticky and builds up, causing problems in many of the body's organs, especially the lungs and pancreas. This disease results in problems with breathing, lung disease, nutrition, digestion, growth, and development.

cystic fibrosis–related diabetes (SYS-tick FY-bro-sis REE-lay-ted DY-uh-beet-eez): a unique form of diabetes that develops in people with cystic fibrosis and has features of both type 1 and type 2 diabetes. This disease substantially lowers survival rates and is frequently diagnosed in people with cystic fibrosis aged 18–21 years. ABBREV.: CFRD.

D

DASH eating plan (dash eet-ing plan): an eating plan based on the one used in the DASH (Dietary Approaches to Stop Hypertension) study, which was prescribed for people with hypertension. This meal plan focuses on limiting intake of saturated fat and cholesterol while increasing intake of foods rich in nutrients that are expected to lower blood pressure, such as minerals (e.g., potassium, calcium, and magnesium), protein, and fiber.

dawn phenomenon (dawhn feh-NAH-meh-nun): the early-morning (4 a.m. to 8 a.m.) rise in blood glucose level.

deductible (DEE-duck-tih-bul): a set amount of money that a person must pay to cover medical care expenses before the insurance company begins paying.

dehydration (dee-hy-DRAY-shun): the loss of too much body fluid through frequent urinating, sweating, diarrhea, or vomiting.

deoxyribonucleic acid (DEE-ox-ee-RY-bow-noo-clay-ic ass-id): a molecule inside the nucleus of cells that carries genetic information and passes it from one generation to the next; the building block of heredity and genes. ABBREV.: DNA.

dermatologist (dur-MAH-tall-uh-jist): a doctor who specializes in diagnosing and treating problems of the skin and hair.

dermopathy (dur-MAH-puh-thee): disease of the skin.

desensitization (dee-sens-ih-tiz-AY-shun): a way to reduce or stop a response, such as an allergic reaction. For example, if someone has an allergic reaction to something, the doctor gives the person a very small amount of the substance to increase one's tolerance. Over a period of time, larger doses are given until the person is taking the full dose. This is one way to help the body get used to the full dose and to prevent the allergic reaction.

detemir insulin (det-eh-meer or det-eh-mer IN-suh-lin): a long-acting insulin analog used to provide a basal or background insulin level. B.N.: Levemir.

dextrose (DECKS-trohs): SYN.: glucose.

diabetes burnout (DY-uh-beet-eez bern-owt): a condition that often affects people with diabetes in which the burdens and constant requirements of diabetes self-management eventually cause the patient to become overwhelmed and frustrated, resulting in lost motivation. People suffering from diabetes burnout often feel defeated by diabetes or angry about having diabetes and try to avoid or cease diabetes care.

Diabetes Control and Complications Trial (DY-uh-beet-eez kon-trol and kom-plih-kay-shuns try-ul): a study by the National Institute of Diabetes and Digestive and Kidney Diseases, conducted from 1983 to 1993 in people with type 1 diabetes. The study showed that intensive therapy compared to conventional therapy significantly helped prevent or delay diabetes complications. Intensive therapy included multiple daily insulin injections or the use of an insulin pump with multiple blood glucose readings each day. The study followed the incidence and prevalence of complications, including diabetic retinopathy, neuropathy, and nephropathy. ABBREV.: DCCT.

diabetes education (DY-uh-beet-eez ed-joo-kay-shun): a program or general curriculum that aims to teach people with diabetes how to address and care for the daily demands of a chronic disease like diabetes. Diabetes education courses and programs usually cover the following topics: general information about diabetes and its treatments, psychological adjustments to life with diabetes, setting goals and solving problems, setting and following a meal plan, increasing exercise, blood glucose monitoring, managing sick days, and identifying and preventing complications.

diabetes educator (DY-uh-beet-eez ed-joo-kay-tor): a health care professional who teaches people who have diabetes how to manage their diabetes. Some diabetes educators are certified diabetes educators (CDEs). Diabetes educators are found in hospitals, physician offices, managed-care organizations, home health care, and other settings.

diabetes insipidus (DY-uh-beet-eez in-SIP-ih-dus): a condition characterized by frequent and heavy urination, excessive thirst, and an overall feeling of weakness. This condition may be caused by a defect in the pituitary gland or in the kidney. In diabetes insipidus, blood glucose levels are normal.

diabetes mellitus (DY-uh-beet-eez MEL-ih-tus): a condition characterized by hyperglycemia resulting from the body's inability to use blood glucose for energy. In type 1 diabetes, the pancreas no longer makes insulin and therefore blood glucose cannot enter the cells to be used for energy. In type 2 diabetes, either the pancreas does not make enough insulin or the body is unable to use insulin correctly.

Diabetes Prevention Program (DY-uh-beet-eez pree-ven-shun pro-gram): a study by the National Institute of Diabetes and Digestive and Kidney Diseases conducted from 1998 to 2001 in people at high risk of developing type 2 diabetes. All study participants had impaired glucose tolerance, also called pre-diabetes, and were overweight. The study showed that people who lost 5–7% of their body weight through a low-fat, low-calorie diet and moderate exercise (usually walking for 30 minutes 5 days a week) reduced their risk of getting type 2 diabetes by 58%. Participants who received treatment with metformin reduced their risk of getting type 2 diabetes by 31%. ABBREV.: DPP.

diabetic coma (DY-uh-beh-tick KOH-mah): a coma that results from diabetic ketoacidosis or hyperosmolar hyperglycemic syndrome.

diabetic diarrhea (DY-uh-beh-tick dy-uh-REE-uh): loose stools, fecal incontinence, or both that result from an overgrowth of bacteria in the small intestine and from diabetic neuropathy in the intestines. This nerve damage can also result in constipation.

diabetic ketoacidosis (DY-uh-beh-tick KEY-toe-ass-ih-DOH-sis): an emergency condition in which extreme hyperglycemia, along with a severe lack of insulin, results in the breakdown of body fat for energy and an accumulation of ketones in the blood and urine. Signs are nausea, vomiting, stomach pain, fruity odor on the breath, and rapid (Kussmaul) breathing. If left untreated, it can lead to coma and death. ABBREV.: DKA.

diabetic mastopathy (DY-uh-beh-tick mass-tah-puh-thee): a rare fibrous breast condition occurring in women, and sometimes men, with long-standing diabetes. The lumps are not malignant and can be surgically removed, although they often recur.

diabetic myelopathy (DY-uh-beh-tick my-eh-LAH-puh-thee): damage to the spinal cord that is found in some people with diabetes.

diabetic neuropathy (DY-uh-beh-tick ne-ROP-uh-thee): neuropathy that arises as a complication of diabetes. ABBREV.: DN.

diabetic retinopathy (DY-uh-beh-tick REH-tih-NOP-uh-thee): retinopathy that arises as a complication of diabetes; damage to the small blood vessels in the retina and subsequent loss of vision can result.

diabetogenic (DY-uh-beh-toh-JEN-ic): anything that causes diabetes.

diabetologist (DY-uh-beh-TAHL-uh-jist): a doctor who specializes in treating people with diabetes.

diagnosis (DY-ug-NO-sis): the determination of a disease from its signs and symptoms.

dialysis (dy-AL-ih-sis): the process of cleaning waste from the blood by filtering it through artificial methods, thus restoring kidney function; prescribed for people whose kidneys have failed as a result of end-stage renal disease. Because nephropathy is a complication of diabetes, people with diabetes can be at risk of having to undergo dialysis. The two major forms of dialysis are hemodialysis and peritoneal dialysis.

diet (DY-et): **1.** the food and drink that a person normally consumes in day-to-day life. **2.** a meal plan in which a person eats or drinks less for a special reason, often to lose weight or to meet the requirements of a disease such as diabetes. **3.** a food or drink that has a reduced amount of calories or certain other nutrients.

dietary fiber (DY-eh-tair-ee FY-bur): fiber contained in the diet, consisting of both soluble and insoluble fiber. General recommendations are for 25–30 grams of fiber per day.

Dietary Reference Intake (DY-eh-tair-ee ref-er-ens in-tayke): the compilation of four indexes of dietary intake that can be used to evaluate or plan diets for individuals and groups; developed by the U.S. Food and Nutrition Board of the National Academy of Sciences beginning in the early 1990s to replace the aging Recommended Dietary Allowances. The four reference values that compose the Dietary Reference Intake are Recommended Dietary Allowance, Adequate Intake, Tolerable Upper Intake Level, and Estimated Average Requirement. ABBREV.: DRI.

dietitian (DY-eh-TIH-shun): a health care professional who advises people about meal planning, weight control, and diabetes management. A registered dietitian (RD) has more training.

dilated eye exam (DY-lay-ted EYE ecks-am): a test done by an eye care specialist in which the pupil (the black center) of the eye is temporarily enlarged with eye drops in order to allow the specialist to more easily see the inside of the eye.

dipeptidyl peptidase-IV (DY-pep-tid-ill pep-tih-dayz fore): an enzyme associated with glucose metabolism. Specifically, it is responsible for

A–E

decreasing the effectiveness and action of incretins such as glucagon-like peptide-1. SYN.: dipeptidyl peptidase-4. ABBREV.: DPP-4 or DPP-IV.

dipeptidyl peptidase-IV inhibitor (DY-pep-tid-ill pep-tih-dayz fore in-hib-it-or): a class of oral hypoglycemic agents that blocks the action of dipeptidyl peptidase-IV. By blocking the action of dipeptidyl peptidase-IV, the action of glucagon-like peptide-1 is not inhibited, allowing the secretion of more insulin to counteract high blood glucose levels. *Ex.*: vildagliptin, sitagliptin.

distal symmetric polyneuropathy (dis-tull sim-et-rick pah-lee-ne-ROP-uh-thee): SYN.: peripheral neuropathy.

diuretic (DY-ur-eh-tick): any substance that increases the production and elimination of urine.

D-phenylalanine derivative (dee-fen-ihl-AL-ah-neen): a class of oral medicine for type 2 diabetes that lowers blood glucose levels by helping the pancreas make more insulin right after meals. G.N.: nateglinide.

Dupuytren's contracture (doo-PWEE-trenz kon-TRACK-chur): a condition associated with diabetes in which the fingers and the palm of the hand thicken and shorten, causing the fingers to curve inward.

Durable Medical Equipment company (der-ah-buhl med-ih-cull ee-kwip-ment kom-pan-ee): a company that sells or rents medical supplies, such as blood glucose meters and test strips, and larger medical equipment, such as hospital beds, wheelchairs, respiratory equipment, and home care items, to the public. Such companies sometimes offer training in the supplies they offer and may have case workers who can help with paperwork. ABBREV.: DME company.

dyslipidemia (dis-lip-ID-eem-ee-uh): abnormal lipid levels, usually referring to high levels of LDL cholesterol, low levels of HDL cholesterol, and/or high levels of triglycerides.

E

eating disorder (eet-ing dis-or-der): a syndrome in which a person eats in a way that disturbs physical, mental, and psychological health; can lead to unpredictable blood glucose levels and diabetes complications. *Ex.*: anorexia nervosa and bulimia.

edema (eh-DEE-muh): swelling caused by excess fluid in the body.

Edmonton protocol (ED-mon-tun PRO-toe-call): a method of islet transplantation first conducted by Drs. James Shapiro, Jonathan Lakey, and Edmond Ryan at the University of Alberta Hospital in the 1990s.

1,800 rule (ATE-teen hun-dred rool): a guideline used by health care professionals to calculate how much one unit of a rapid-acting insulin analog (such as lispro, aspart, or glulisine) will lower blood glucose levels. It is calculated as such: divide 1,800 by the total daily dose of rapid-acting insulin analog in units. The result is the estimated amount that one unit of insulin will lower blood glucose levels.

electromyography (ee-LEK-troh-my-AH-gruh-fee): a test used to detect nerve function; measures the electrical activity generated by muscles.

endocrine gland (EN-doh-krin gland): a group of specialized cells that release hormones into the blood. *Ex.*: the islets in the pancreas, which secrete insulin, are endocrine glands.

endocrinologist (EN-doh-krih-NAH-luh-jist): a doctor who treats people who have endocrine gland problems, such as diabetes.

endocrinology (EN-doh-krih-NAH-luh-gee): the study of hormones produced by the body.

endocrinopathy (EN-doh-krin-AH-puh-thee): disease of the endocrine glands.

end-stage renal disease (end-stay-jeh REE-nal dih-zeez): SYN.: kidney failure. ABBREV.: ESRD.

enzyme (EN-zime): protein made by the body that brings about a chemical reaction; for example, the enzymes produced by the gut to aid digestion.

epidemiology (ep-ih-DEEM-ee-ah-LUH-gee): the study of disease patterns in humans that deals with how many people have that particular disease, where the population is located, how many new cases of the disease develop, and how the disease is controlled.

erectile dysfunction (ee-REK-tile dis-FUNK-shun): the inability to get or maintain an erection for sexual activity; a complication of diabetes that is usually treated with medication. SYN.: impotence. ABBREV.: ED.

erythrocyte (ih-rith-RO-syte): SYN.: red blood cell.

Estimated Average Requirement (EH-stih-may-ted AV-rihj REE-kwi-ur-ment): one of the four reference values of the Dietary Reference Intake; estimates the amount of a nutrient needed to meet the requirement of half of the healthy individuals in an age-group and gender group; used to assess dietary adequacy and as the basis for the Recommended Dietary Allowance. ABBREV.: EAR.

A–E

estrogen (eh-STRO-jen): female hormone secreted primarily by the ovaries (also by the testes in men) that is active in the menstrual cycle and other female characteristics; during the menstrual cycle in some women, estrogen can cause blood glucose levels to fluctuate.

euglycemia (you-gly-SEEM-ee-uh): a normal level of glucose in the blood.

exchange list (EKS-chaynj lihst): one of several approaches for diabetes meal planning. Foods are categorized into seven groups based on nutritional content and a standardized serving size: starch/bread, meat and meat substitutes, vegetables, fruits, milk, fat, and other carbohydrates. Following exchange lists allows for the substitution of one food item for another food item but keeps the nutritional value of the diet fixed.

exclusive provider organization (ecks-clew-siv PRO-vi-dur or-gan-ih-zay-shun): a type of managed-care organization; specifically, a type of preferred provider organization in which individual members use assigned physicians rather than having a choice of a variety of providers. ABBREV.: EPO.

exenatide (ECKS-en-ah-TIED): the first in a class of drugs called incretin mimetics used for the treatment of type 2 diabetes. Exenatide is a synthetic version of exendin-4, a naturally occurring hormone that was first isolated from the saliva of the Gila monster, a lizard. Exenatide works to lower blood glucose levels primarily by increasing insulin secretion and is administered by injection. Because it only has this effect in the presence of elevated blood glucose levels, it does not tend to increase the risk of hypoglycemia when taken alone, but can when used in combination therapy. The primary side effect is nausea, which tends to improve over time. B.N.: Byetta.

exercise physiologist (ecks-er-size fizz-EE-ahl-uh-jist): a specialist trained in the science of exercise and body conditioning who can help patients plan a safe, effective exercise program.

eye doctor (AYE dock-tor): an optometrist.

F

fad diet (fad DY-et): a diet (usually for weight loss) that promises unrealistically quick and fantastic results and enjoys widespread popularity for a short time.

fasting (fast-ing): going without food or drink for a prescribed amount of time.

fasting plasma glucose test (fast-ing PLAZ-muh GLOO-kose test): a test that checks a person's blood glucose level after the person has not eaten for 8–12 hours (usually overnight); used to diagnose pre-diabetes and diabetes and to monitor blood glucose levels in people with diabetes. If diabetes is not diagnosed, but blood glucose levels are still abnormal, impaired fasting glucose is diagnosed. SYN.: fasting blood glucose test. ABBREV.: FPG.

fat (fat): **1.** One of the main nutrients in food. Foods that provide fat are butter, margarine, salad dressing, oil, nuts, meat, poultry, fish, and some dairy products. **2.** Any of the different kinds of fat found in food, including monounsaturated fat, omega-3 fatty acid, polyunsaturated fat, saturated fat, and trans fatty acid. **3.** Excess calories are stored as adipose tissue (also called body fat), which provides the body with a reserve supply of energy, keeps it insulated, and cushions it. **4.** When in the body, particularly in the bloodstream, it is often called a lipid or blood fat.

fee-for-service health care (fee-for-ser-viss helth kair): a type of health care insurance in which the insurance company pays for the services and costs incurred by the insured person. The insured person has the flexibility to select the hospital, clinic, and/or doctors; however, the insurance company will often not pay 100% of the medical expenses incurred. People belonging to such a plan can expect to pay a monthly fee (or premium), a deductible, and, if applicable, co-insurance. The most commonly known providers of this form of health insurance are Blue Cross and Blue Shield.

fiber (FY-bur): SYN.: dietary fiber.

15-gram/15-minute rule (fif-TEEN gram/fif-TEEN min-it rool): a method of treating hypoglycemia;

when blood glucose levels are low, the patient takes a 15-gram carbohydrate source (such as a glucose tablet, 1/2 cup juice, or 1 cup non-fat milk), waits 15 minutes, and then checks levels again. If blood glucose levels remain low, the patient repeats the process until the levels optimize.

1,500 rule (fif-TEEN hun-dred rool): a guideline used by health care professionals to calculate how much one unit of regular (short-acting) insulin will lower blood glucose levels. It is calculated as such: divide 1,500 by the total daily dose of regular insulin in units. The result is the estimated amount that one unit of regular insulin will lower blood glucose levels.

50/50 insulin (fif-TEE fif-TEE IN-suh-lin): premixed insulin that is 50% intermediate-acting insulin and 50% short-acting (regular) insulin.

F.I.T.T. Principle (fit prin-sih-puhl): a guideline designed to help people create and follow a healthy, safe exercise plan; stands for Frequency, Intensity, Time, and Type. Frequency refers to how often a person exercises per week. Intensity refers to the level of exertion achieved during exercise. Time refers to the amount of time spent at the target intensity level. Type refers to the types of exercise followed, including aerobic exercise, strength training, and flexibility exercise, and encourages diversity in the exercise routine, which reduces the risk of injury.

504 Plan (five-oh-for plan): a plan developed to meet the requirements of a federal law that prohibits discrimination against people with disabilities, Section 504 of the Rehabilitation Act of 1973. Section 504 applies to all public schools and to private schools that receive federal funds. A 504 Plan sets out an agreement to ensure that the student has the same access to education as other children and can be used to make sure that the student, the parents/guardians, and school personnel understand their responsibilities and to prepare for possible problem situations. It may be developed as a result of a request by the school, a request by the parents/guardians, or in response to a problem with the student's care at school.

flexibility exercise (FLEX-ih-bill-ih-TEE ecks-er-size): any of the many physical activities that increases the body's flexibility. SYN. stretching.

fluorescein angiography (fluh-RESS-ee-in an-gee-AH-grah-fee): a test to examine blood vessels in the eye; done by injecting dye into an arm vein and then taking photos as the dye goes through the eye's blood vessels.

F–J

focal neuropathy (FOH-cull ne-ROP-uh-thee): a condition due to damage to a single nerve or group of nerves that usually goes away in 2 weeks to 18 months; caused either by blockage of a blood vessel that supplies the nerve or nerves with blood or by a pinched nerve. *Ex.*: carpal tunnel syndrome.

food diary (food DY-er-ee): a logbook in which a person records every bit of food and drink consumed over a set period of time (usually a number of weeks); used to help create a personalized meal plan; often also records physical activity and blood glucose levels.

food label (food LAY-bul): a Nutrition Facts label.

food pyramid (food PEER-ah-mid): a visual representation of a balanced, healthy diet, often broken into different sections representing different types of foods. In 2005, the U.S. Department of Agriculture radically revised the food pyramid from one with four or six food groups to a more personalized food pyramid that breaks daily calorie consumption into percentages of each different type of food, including grains, vegetables, fruits, milk, meat and beans, and oils and discretionary calories. This new pyramid also compensates for body type, age, sex, and physical activity level.

Framingham Heart Study (FRAME-ing-ham hart stuh-dee): a cardiovascular health study based in Framingham, Massachusetts, that began in 1948. The original study group consisted of 5,209 adults from Framingham and has continued through the decades by studying the children of the original study subjects. It is currently on its third generation of study subjects. Most of the knowledge concerning heart disease that we consider commonplace, such as the effects of diet, exercise, and common medications (e.g., aspirin) on heart health, are based on the data collected from this important study. It is a project of the National Heart, Lung, and Blood Institute in collaboration with Boston University (begun in 1971).

free radical (free RAD-ih-cull): a naturally occurring, chemically reactive atom or molecule with a free or unpaired electron that is essential in many biological processes; its high reactivity can lead to cell damage, including apoptosis; may be associated with a number of conditions and diseases, including atherosclerosis, cancer, cardiovascular disease, and emphysema.

fructosamine test (frook-TOH-sah-meen test): a measure of the number of blood glucose molecules linked to protein molecules in the blood; provides information on average blood glucose levels for the past 2–3 weeks; often used in patients who cannot undergo the A1C test, e.g., a person with anemia.

fructose (FROOK-tohs): a sugar that occurs naturally in fruits and honey; has 4 calories per gram.

G

gangrene (GANG-green): the death of body tissue, most often caused by a lack of blood flow and infection; can lead to amputation.

gastric bypass surgery (ga-strick by-pass sur-jur-ee): a bariatric surgical procedure in which the stomach is made smaller and digestion bypasses part of the small intestine; often done to help patients lose large amounts of body weight, particularly in those with a body mass index over 40 kg/m^2.

gastric inhibitory polypeptide (ga-strick in-hib-ih-tor-ee pah-lee-PEP-tide): an incretin that stimulates insulin secretion. Also called glucose-dependent insulinotropic peptide. ABBREV.: GIP.

gastroparesis (gas-tro-puh-REE-sis): a form of neuropathy that affects the stomach. Digestion of food may be incomplete or delayed, resulting in nausea, vomiting, or bloating, making blood glucose levels difficult to control.

gene (jeen): the basic biological unit of heredity composed of a sequence of DNA.

gene therapy (jeen thair-uh-pee): an approach to treating diseases by changing or altering the genes that cause the disease.

genetics (JEN-eh-ticks): study of how particular qualities or traits are transmitted from parents to children; study of heredity.

gestational diabetes mellitus (jes-TAY-shun-ul DY-uh-beet-eez MEL-ih-tus): a type of diabetes that develops only during pregnancy and usually disappears upon delivery, but increases the risk that the mother will later develop diabetes; managed with meal planning, physical activity, and sometimes insulin. ABBREV.: GDM.

gingivitis (JIN-jih-VY-tis): a condition of the gums characterized by inflammation and bleeding.

gland (gland): a group of cells that secretes substances, such as hormones.

glargine insulin (GLAR-jeen IN-suh-lin): a long-acting basal insulin analog that, on average,

F–J

starts to lower blood glucose levels within 1 hour after injection and keeps working evenly for about 24 hours after injection. B.N.: Lantus.

glaucoma (glaw-KOH-mah): a disease that damages the optic nerve, often caused by an increase of pressure inside the eye. Can lead to a loss of vision.

glimepiride (gly-MEH-per-ide): an oral medicine used to treat type 2 diabetes that belongs to the class of medicines called sulfonylureas. B.N.: Amaryl.

glipizide (GLIH-pih-zide): an oral medicine used to treat type 2 diabetes that belongs to the class of medicines called sulfonylureas. B.N.: Glucotrol, Glucotrol XL.

glomerular filtration rate (glo-MEHR-yoo-lur fil-TRAY-shun rayte): a measure of the ability of the kidneys to filter and remove waste products.

glomerulus (glo-MEHR-yoo-lus): a tiny set of looping blood vessels in the kidney where the blood is filtered and waste products are removed.

glucagon (GLOO-kah-gahn): a hormone produced by the alpha cells in the pancreas that raises blood glucose levels. An injectable form of glucagon, available by prescription, may be used to treat severe hypoglycemia.

glucagon-like peptide-1 (GLOO-kah-gahn-lyke pep-tide wan): an incretin that increases insulin secretion from the pancreas, a characteristic that can make it helpful in treating diabetes. ABBREV.: GLP-1.

glucocorticoid (GLOO-koh-cor-tih-coyd): a compound that belongs to the family of compounds called corticosteroids; affects metabolism and has anti-inflammatory and immunosuppressive effects; may be produced naturally (hormones) or synthetically (drugs).

glucometer (GLOO-koh-mee-tur): SYN.: blood glucose meter.

glucose (GLOO-kose): one of the simplest forms of sugar; a simple sugar found in blood that serves as the body's main source of energy. SYN.: dextrose.

glucose-dependent insulinotropic peptide (GLOO-kose-DEE-pen-dent IN-suh-lin-oh-troe-pick pep-tide): an incretin that stimulates insulin secretion. Also called gastric inhibitory polypeptide. ABBREV.: GIP.

glucose metabolism (GLOO-kose met-ab-ohl-izm): the process by which glucose is converted to energy.

glucose tablet (GLOO-kose tab-let): a chewable tablet made of pure glucose; used to treat hypoglycemia.

glucose tolerance test (GLOO-kose tohl-er-ENTS test): a test used to determine whether a person has abnormal blood glucose levels, including diabetes; usually, after a set period of fasting, a person is given a drink with glucose in it and then blood glucose levels are tested at different times to see where they stand. There are two types of this test: the fasting plasma glucose test and the oral glucose tolerance test. ABBREV.: GTT.

glulisine insulin (GLOO-lih-seen IN-suh-lin): a rapid-acting insulin analog. On average, gluli-

F–J

sine insulin starts to lower blood glucose levels within 15 minutes after injection. It has its strongest effect 1 to 1 1/2 hours after injection but keeps working for 3 hours after injection. B.N.: Apidra.

glutamic acid decarboxylase antibody (GLOO-tam-ick ass-id DEE-car-box-ee-layze AN-tee-bod-ee): an autoantibody that attacks glutamic acid decarboxylase (GAD), a protein made by the beta cells in the pancreas. It is thought that the similarity between GAD and the Coxsackie B4 virus may influence the production of these antibodies, which may lead to the development of type 1 diabetes. ABBREV.: GAD antibody.

gluten (GLOO-ten): a type of protein found in wheat, rye, barley, possibly oats, and some other grains, including most common flours; can also be found in certain medications and in some store-bought items (e.g., some brands of soy sauce).

gluten-free diet (GLOO-ten free DY-et): the prescribed treatment for celiac disease, in which a person has no gluten in his or her daily diet.

gluten-sensitive enteropathy (GLOO-ten sens-ih-tiv en-ter-ah-puth-ee): SYN.: celiac disease.

glyburide (GLY-buh-ride): an oral medicine used to treat type 2 diabetes that belongs to the class of medicines called sulfonylureas. B.N.: DiaBeta, Glynase PresTab, Micronase.

glycated hemoglobin (gly-KAY-ted HEE-mo-glo-bin): SYN.: glycosylated hemoglobin.

glycemia (gly-SEE-me-uh): the concentration of glucose in the blood.

glycemic index (gly-SEE-mik in-decks): a ranking of carbohydrate-containing foods, based on the food's effect on blood glucose levels compared with a standard reference food.

glycogen (GLY-koh-jen): the form of glucose found in the liver and muscles.

glycosylated hemoglobin (gly-KOH-sih-lated HEE-mo-glo-bin): a form of hemoglobin to which glucose has joined; in people with diabetes, the amount of glycosylated hemoglobin is increased and can be measured to determine average blood glucose levels over a certain period of time (see A1C test). SYN.: glycated hemoglobin, hemoglobin A1C, glycohemoglobin. ABBREV.: GHb, HbA_{1c}.

glycosuria (gly-koh-SOOR-ee-ah): the presence of glucose in the urine.

gram (gram): a unit of weight in the metric system; 1 ounce equals 28 grams.

group insurance (GROOP in-shur-ens): a health insurance policy in which groups of employees (and sometimes dependents) are covered under a single policy or contract that is issued by an employer.

H

HbA_{1c} (AYTCH-bee-AY-wan-see): SYN.: glycosylated hemoglobin.

health care team (helth kair teem): a group of health care professionals who work with a patient to help in the care of a chronic disease (a process called team management); often used in the treatment of diabetes and may include a doctor, diabetes educator, dietitian, exercise physiologist, optometrist, podiatrist, and pharmacist.

Health Insurance Portability and Accountability Act (helth in-shur-ens por-tah-bil-it-ee and ah-cownt-uh-bil-ih-tee act): a law enacted in 1996 under which insurers and employers may not make insurance rules that discriminate against workers because of their health. All workers eligible for a certain health insurance plan must be offered enrollment at the same price. ABBREV.: HIPAA.

health maintenance organization (helth MAYN-ten-ents or-gan-ih-zay-shun): a type of managed-care organization that is a prepaid health insurance plan; members pay a monthly premium for comprehensive care from the organization's hospitals, offices, and staff, which are only available to members. ABBREV.: HMO.

heart attack (hart uh-tack): an interruption in the blood supply to the heart because of narrowed or blocked blood vessels, causing muscle damage and sometimes death. SYN.: myocardial infarction.

heart disease (hart dih-zeez): a condition that affects the heart muscle or the blood vessels of the heart.

heart rate (hart rayte): the number of times the heart beats in 1 minute; pulse.

hemoglobin (HEE-mo-glo-bin): the part of a red blood cell that carries oxygen to the cells; when it joins with the glucose in the bloodstream, it is called glycosylated hemoglobin or HbA_{1c}.

hemodialysis (HEE-mo-dy-AL-ih-sis): a type of dialysis in which a machine called a dialyzer is used to filter the blood in place of kidneys that have failed as a result of end-stage renal disease; it is usually a lengthy procedure, requiring 3–4 hours at a time, and is performed three times a week.

hemorrhage (hem-OR-idge): sudden and abnormal bleeding, usually with a great deal of blood, that occurs either inside or outside of the body.

heredity (HER-ed-it-ee): the passing of a trait from parent to child.

high blood pressure (HI blud preh-shure): SYN.: hypertension.

high-density lipoprotein cholesterol (HI-den-SIH-tee LIPE-oh-PRO-teen kuh-LESS-tuh-rawl): a fat found in the blood that takes extra cholesterol in the blood to the liver for removal; often called "good" or "healthy" cholesterol. ABBREV.: HDL cholesterol.

honeymoon phase (hun-EE-moon faze): a brief remission of type 1 diabetes that sometimes occurs soon after the diagnosis of diabetes is made. During this time, the pancreas may still secrete some insulin, but over time, this secretion will stop. This condition can last weeks, months, a year, or longer.

hormone (HORE-mown): a chemical produced in one part of the body and released into the blood to trigger or regulate particular functions of the body. Synthetic hormones, made for use as medicines, can be the same or different from those made in the body. *Ex.*: insulin is a hormone made in the pancreas that tells other cells when to use glucose for energy.

human leukocyte antigen (HEW-man LEW-co-site an-TIH-jen): a protein located on the surface of the cell that helps the immune system identify whether the cell belongs to the self or is a foreign object; if it improperly identifies a cell as a foreign object, then an autoimmune attack is triggered, in which the immune system attacks the cells of the body. Particular types of the human leukocyte antigen are more common in people with diabetes, which suggests that there is a connection between the protein and the disease. ABBREV.: HLA.

hyperglycemia (HY-per-gly-SEE-mee-uh): a condition characterized by excessively high blood glucose levels; signs include excessive thirst (polydipsia), excessive urination (polyuria), and excessive hunger (polyphagia).

hyperinsulinemia (HY-per-IN-suh-lih-NEE-mee-uh): a condition in which the level of insulin in the blood is higher than normal; caused by overproduction of insulin by the body; related to insulin resistance.

F–J

hyperlipidemia (HY-per-lih-pih-DEE-mee-uh): higher-than-normal fat and cholesterol levels in the blood.

hypernatremia (HY-per-nuh-TREE-me-uh): a condition characterized by excessive amounts of sodium in the blood, usually due to a lack of fluid in the body; can be an indicator of diabetes insipidus.

hyperosmolar hyperglycemic syndrome (HY-per-oz-MOH-lur HY-per-gly-SEE-mik sin-drohm): an emergency condition in which one's blood glucose level is very high, but ketones are not present in the blood or urine. If left untreated, it can lead to coma or death. SYN.: hyperosmolar hyperglycemic nonketotic syndrome (HHNS). ABBREV.: HHS.

hypertension (HY-per-TEN-shun): a condition present when blood flows through the blood vessels with a force greater than normal, thus straining the heart, damaging blood vessels, and increasing the risk of heart attack, stroke, and kidney disease. SYN.: high blood pressure. ABBREV.: HTN.

F–J

hyperthyroidism (HY-per-THI-royd-ism): **1.** a condition marked by an overactive thyroid gland that produces too much thyroid hormone. **2.** the condition that results from an overactive thyroid gland, which usually includes enlargement of the thyroid gland, rapid heart rate, and hypertension; this can make blood glucose management difficult in people with diabetes.

hypertrophy (hy-PER-truh-fee): SYN.: lipohypertrophy.

hypoglycemia (hy-po-gly-SEE-mee-uh): a condition characterized by abnormally low blood glucose levels, usually less than 70 mg/dl; signs include hunger, nervousness, shakiness, perspiration, dizziness, light-headedness, sleepiness, and confusion. If left untreated, hypoglycemia may lead to unconsciousness. SYN.: insulin reaction.

hypoglycemia unawareness (hy-po-gly-SEE-mee-uh un-uh-WARE-ness): a state in which a person does not feel or recognize the symptoms of hypoglycemia.

F–J

hyponatremia (HY-poh-nuh-TREE-me-uh): an abnormally low level of sodium in the blood; this dangerous condition can be caused by burns, vomiting, diarrhea, use of diuretics (especially thiazide diuretics), kidney disease, and congestive heart failure.

hypotension (hy-poh-TEN-shun): low blood pressure or a sudden drop in blood pressure; may occur when a person rises quickly from a seated or reclined position, which can cause dizziness or fainting.

hypothyroidism (HY-poh-THI-royd-ism): **1.** a condition in which the thyroid gland produces too little thyroid hormone. **2.** the condition that results from an underactive thyroid gland, which usually includes fatigue, weight gain, constipation, dry skin, and sensitivity to the cold; this can make blood glucose management difficult in people with diabetes.

I

immune system (ih-MYOON SIS-tem): the body's system for protecting itself from viruses and bacteria or any "foreign" substances.

immunity (ih-MYOON-ih-tee): a state in which the body can resist a certain disease. It is developed or gained against only individual diseases and lasts for varying amounts of time.

immunization (ih-MYOON-ih-zay-shun): **1.** the process used to create immunity (or resistance) to a specific disease. **2.** SYN.: vaccination. [*Usage*: both "immunization" and "vaccination" are often used interchangeably.] When used in this sense: a process by which an individual is exposed to an agent (called an immunogen) that is designed to provoke an attack by the immune system against that particular agent. If the immune response is successful, the body will be protected against that disease in the future. This procedure works because the human immune system can develop the ability to quickly respond to a disease after it has been exposed to it before.

immunosuppressant (ih-MYOON-oh-suh-PRESS-unt): a drug that suppresses the natural immune responses, i.e., causes immunosuppression; given to transplant patients to prevent organ rejection or to patients with autoimmune disease.

immunosuppression (ih-MYOON-oh-suh-PRESS-shun): the condition in which the body's immune system and its ability to fight infections or disease is inhibited or stopped; may be caused by a disease (such as HIV) or intentionally with immunosuppressants to prevent organ rejection in transplant patients.

impaired fasting glucose (im-PAIR-d FAST-ing GLOO-kose): a condition in which a fasting plasma glucose test, taken after 8–12 hours of fasting, shows a blood glucose level that is higher than normal but not high enough for a diagnosis of diabetes. People with impaired fasting glucose are at increased risk for developing type 2 diabetes. Also called pre-diabetes. ABBREV.: IFG.

impaired glucose tolerance (im-PAIR-d GLOO-kose tohl-er-ENTS): a condition in which an oral glucose tolerance test shows a blood glucose level higher than normal but not high enough for a diagnosis of diabetes. People with impaired glucose tolerance are at increased risk for developing type 2 diabetes. Also called pre-diabetes, borderline diabetes (OBS.), subclinical diabetes (OBS.), chemical diabetes (OBS.), and latent diabetes (OBS.). ABBREV.: IGT.

implantable insulin pump (im-PLAN-tuh-bull IN-suh-lin pump): an insulin pump that is placed inside the body to deliver insulin in response to remote-control commands from the user.

impotence (IM-po-tents): SYN.: erectile dysfunction; a complication of diabetes.

incidence (IN-sih-dints): a measure of how often a disease occurs; the number of new cases of a disease among a certain group of people for a certain period of time.

incontinence (in-KON-tih-nents): loss of bladder or bowel control; the involuntary loss of urine or feces.

incretin (in-CREE-tin): a type of hormone that causes an increase in the amount of insulin released from the beta cells of the islets of Langerhans after eating, even before blood glucose levels become elevated.

incretin mimetic (in-CREE-tin MIME-eh-tick): a class of medications used to treat type 2 diabetes; functions by mimicking (or reproducing) the blood glucose–lowering effects of the naturally occurring incretin hormone. *Ex.*: exenatide.

Individualized Education Program (in-div-id-you-uhl-IZE-d ed-JOO-kay-shun PRO-gram): under the Individuals with Disabilities in Education Act, a diabetes management plan collaboratively developed by school personnel and the parents of a child with diabetes that describes the steps taken to ensure that the student has the same opportunities to participate in all academic and school-sponsored activities while maintaining the student's health; often, this program is more specific than a 504 Plan with regard to the student's academic needs. ABBREV.: IEP.

Individuals with Disabilities in Education Act (in-div-id-you-uls with dis-ah-bil-ih-tees in ed-JOO-kay-shun act): a law that guarantees free public education to children with disabilities; children whose diabetes aversely affects their ability to learn generally qualify for protection under this law and often receive an Individualized Education Program. ABBREV.: IDEA.

infection (in-FECKT-shun): the state that exists when the body is invaded by an infectious agent, such as bacteria, fungi, or viruses, possibly resulting in the development of a disease. People with diabetes are at greater risk of infection due to the effect high blood glucose levels have on the effectiveness of white blood cells.

inflammation (in-fluh-MAY-shun): the body's protective response to infection and injury that is characterized in its more serious forms by pain, heat, redness, swelling, and loss of function; scientific research has suggested that inflammation is possibly linked to the development of cardiovascular disease and type 2 diabetes (as investigated through levels of C-reactive protein in the blood).

F–J

inhaled insulin (in-HAY-uld IN-suh-lin): a rapid-acting insulin that comes in powdered form and is administered through a portable device (called an inhaler) that allows a person to breathe in the insulin. B.N.: Exubera.

injection (in-JEK-shun): the process of inserting liquid medication (e.g., insulin) or nutrients into the body with a syringe and needle.

injection site (in-JEK-shun syte): the place on the body where a medication (e.g., insulin) or nutrient is usually injected.

injection site rotation (in-JEK-shun syte ROW-tay-shun): the process of changing between several different places on the body where an injection is administered; prevents the formation of lipodystrophy.

insoluble fiber (in-soll-you-buhl FY-bur): dietary fiber found in the parts of plants that the body cannot digest, such as wheat bran and fruit and vegetable skins; aids in the normal functioning of the digestive system.

insulin (IN-suh-lin): a polypeptide hormone that helps the body use glucose for energy; created by the beta cells of the pancreas. All animals (including humans) require insulin to survive.

insulin adjustment (IN-suh-lin uhd-JUST-ment): the process of changing the amount of insulin a person with diabetes takes based on factors such as meal planning, activity, and blood glucose levels.

insulin analog (IN-suh-lin anna-log): a genetically engineered form of insulin that is derived from the human insulin molecule. An analog acts in much the same way as the body's native insulin, but with some beneficial differences for people with diabetes, such as shorter or longer peaks, shorter or longer durations, increased purity, and reduced risk of allergic reactions. Analogs have been developed to serve as basal insulin or bolus insulin.

insulin autoantibody (IN-suh-lin AN-tee-bod-ee): an autoantibody that attacks insulin, which can make insulin less effective or completely eliminate it altogether. Often the presence of insulin autoantibodies indicates that a person has insulin resistance. The presence of certain strains of insulin antibodies can also indicate an allergic reaction to insulin of varying strengths (this often arises in people who already take insulin to care for diabetes or in those who have taken beef insulin, which is no longer produced in the U.S.). SYN.: insulin antibody, anti-insulin antibody. ABBREV.: IAA.

insulin-dependent diabetes mellitus (IN-suh-lin-DEE-pen-dent DY-uh-beet-eez MEL-ih-tus): OBS.: type 1 diabetes. [*Usage*: so called because of the perception that this particular form of diabetes was the only one that required insulin therapy; with the advent of insulin use in patients with type 2 diabetes, or NIDDM, this term became less useful.] ABBREV.: IDDM.

insulin pen (IN-suh-lin pen): a device for injecting insulin; it resembles a fountain pen and holds replaceable cartridges of insulin; a dial is often used to set the insulin dose; some pens are disposable.

insulin pump (IN-suh-lin pump): an insulin-delivering device about the size of a deck of cards that can be worn on a belt or kept in a pocket.

It carries a reservoir of insulin connected to narrow, flexible plastic tubing that ends with a needle that is inserted just under the skin. Users set the pump to give a basal amount of insulin continuously throughout the day. Pumps also release bolus insulin to cover meals and at times when blood glucose levels are high, based on programming done by the user.

insulin reaction (IN-suh-lin REE-ack-shun): a bodily response to low blood glucose levels. SYN.: hypoglycemia.

insulin receptor (IN-suh-lin REE-sep-tur): an area on the outer part of a cell that allows the cell to bind with insulin in the blood. When the cell and insulin bind, the cell can take glucose from the blood and use it for energy.

insulin resistance (IN-suh-lin REE-sis-tens): a condition characterized by the body's inability to respond to and use the insulin that it produces, meaning that insulin cannot function properly and higher levels of insulin are needed to achieve the same effects. This can result in high blood glucose levels and high levels of insulin in the blood. If allowed to worsen,

F–J

pre-diabetes and type 2 diabetes can develop. Insulin resistance develops in people who have a family history of it, in people who are overweight, and in people who live a sedentary lifestyle. It is also one of the conditions included in the metabolic syndrome.

insulin resistance syndrome (IN-suh-lin REE-sistens sin-drohm): SYN.: metabolic syndrome, Syndrome X.

insulinoma (IN-suh-lih-NOH-mah): a tumor of the beta cells in the pancreas; may cause overproduction of insulin, resulting in hypoglycemia.

intensive therapy (in-TENS-iv thair-uh-pee): a rigorous treatment for diabetes in which blood glucose levels are kept as close to normal as possible through frequent insulin injections or use of an insulin pump; meal planning; adjustment of medicines; and exercise based on frequent results of self-monitoring of blood glucose (SMBG) and frequent contact with a health care team; requires training and dedication on the part of the patient with diabetes, but often results with better health outcomes; increases risk of hypoglycemia; contrast with conventional therapy.

intermediate-acting insulin (IN-ter-meed-EE-et-ackt-ing IN-suh-lin): a type of insulin that starts to lower blood glucose levels within 1–2 hours after injection and has its strongest effect 6–12 hours after injection, depending on the type used. *Ex.*: NPH insulin.

intermittent claudication (IN-ter-MIT-ent CLAW-dih-KAY-shun): pain that comes and goes in the muscles of the leg; often results from a lack of blood supply to the legs and usually happens when walking or exercising.

intramuscular injection (in-trah-MUS-kyoo-lar in-JEK-shun): inserting liquid medication into a muscle with a syringe. *Ex.*: Glucagon may be given by intramuscular injection to treat hypoglycemia.

intravenous (in-trah-VEEN-us): injected directly into a vein. ABBREV.: IV.

ischemia (is-KEE-mee-uh): a complete stoppage or shortage of blood supply to an organ or other body part; can be caused by a variety of situations, including atherosclerosis, hypotension, and tachycardia. If left untreated, it can quickly lead to necrosis of the affected organ or body part.

islet cell (EYE-let sel): any of the many types of cells located in the pancreas that make hormones to help the body break down and use food for energy. SYN.: islets of Langerhans. *Ex.*: alpha cells make glucagon, beta cells make insulin.

islet cell autoantibody (EYE-let sel aw-toe-AN-tih-bod-ee): proteins found in the blood of people newly diagnosed with or who may be developing type 1 diabetes; its presence indicates that the body's immune system has been damaging and killing the beta cells in the pancreas. ABBREV.: ICA.

islet cell transplantation (EYE-let TRANS-plan-tay-shun): a procedure in which islet cells are moved from a donor pancreas into a person whose pancreas has stopped producing insulin; this allows the islet recipient to again begin producing his or her own insulin;

intended as a cure for type 1 diabetes. This is still an experimental procedure that requires the use of immunosuppressants to stop the immune system from rejecting donor islets. An additional difficulty is the small donor pool, meaning that there are not enough potential donor islets available. Sometimes referred to as the Edmonton protocol, a method of conducting this procedure.

islets of Langerhans (EYE-lets of LANG-er-hahns): SYN.: islet cell. Named after German anatomist Paul Langerhans, who discovered them in 1869.

F-J

J

jet injector (JET in-JEK-tur): a device that uses high pressure instead of a needle to propel insulin through the skin and into the body.

juvenile diabetes (JOO-vuh-nile DY-uh-beet-eez): OBS.: type 1 diabetes.

K

ketoacidosis (KEY-toe-ass-ih-DOH-sis): SYN.: diabetic ketoacidosis.

ketone (KEY-tone): a waste product that results from the process of the body breaking down body fat for energy, which is a situation that arises when there is a shortage of insulin. High levels can lead to diabetic ketoacidosis and coma. SYN.: ketone body.

ketonuria (key-toe-NUH-ree-ah): a condition occurring when ketones are present in the urine; a warning sign of diabetic ketoacidosis.

ketosis (key-TOE-sis): an elevated level of ketones in the body, which may lead to diabetic ketoacidosis. Signs of ketosis are nausea, vomiting, and stomach pain.

kidney (KID-nee): the two bean-shaped organs located on both sides of the spine on the lower back that filter wastes from the blood and eliminate it from the body in the form of urine.

kidney failure (KID-nee FAYL-yur): a chronic condition in which the kidneys no longer work properly; resulting in the body retaining fluid and causing harmful wastes to build up inside the body; this life-threatening condition is usually treated with dialysis or a kidney transplant. SYN.: end-stage renal disease.

kilocalorie (KEE-lo-CAL-or-ee): a metric unit that is equal to the amount of heat required to raise the temperature of 1 kilogram of water by 1 degree Celsius; in nutrition, it is used to measure the amount of energy produced by a food. [*Usage*: common use of the word "calorie" (in nutrition) is a shortened version of this term: "kilocalorie."] SYN.: calorie.

Kussmaul breathing (KOOS-mall bree-thing): the rapid, deep, and labored breathing of people who have diabetic ketoacidosis.

L

lactic acidosis (LACK-tic ass-ih-DOH-sis): a serious and possibly fatal condition caused by the build up of lactic acid in the body, which is

K–O

produced when cells burn glucose for energy without enough oxygen; signs are deep and rapid breathing, vomiting, and abdominal pain; may be caused by diabetic ketoacidosis, liver or kidney disease, or some drugs (such as metformin in certain high-risk groups).

lactose (LACK-tose): a type of sugar found in milk and milk products.

lancet (LAN-set): a spring-loaded device used to prick the skin with a small needle in order to obtain a drop of blood for blood glucose monitoring.

K–O

laser surgery treatment (LAY-zer sur-jur-ee TREET-ment): a type of therapy that uses a laser (a strong beam of light) to treat a damaged area; in diabetes, often used to seal damaged blood vessels. *Ex.*: photocoagulation.

latent autoimmune diabetes in adults (LAY-tint AW-tow-ih-MYOON DY-uh-beet-eez in UH-dults): a hereditary autoimmune disease that shares many of the characteristics of type 1 diabetes and develops in adults. ABBREV.: LADA.

latent diabetes (LAY-tint DY-uh-beet-eez): OBS.; SYN.: impaired glucose tolerance.

Lente insulin (LEN-tay IN-suh-lin): an intermediate-acting insulin. On average, it starts to lower blood glucose levels within 1–2 hours after injection and has its strongest effect 8–12 hours after injection but keeps working for 18–24 hours after injection. As of 2005, this insulin is no longer manufactured.

licensed practical nurse (LI-sens-d PRACK-tih-cul nurs): a nurse who has received 1–2 years of training, received certification and licensing from a state authority, and works under the supervision of registered nurses and physicians. Also called licensed vocational nurse (LVN). ABBREV.: LPN.

lifestyle (LYFE-stile): the way a person or group of people lives.

limited joint mobility (LIM-ih-ted joynt MOH-bil-ih-tee): a condition in which the joints swell and the skin of the hand becomes thick, tight, and waxy, making the joints less able to move; may affect the fingers and arms as well as other

K–O

joints in the body; arises in people with type 1 diabetes as a result of microvascular disease or complications. SYN.: cheiroarthropathy. ABBREV.: LJM.

lipid (LIP-id): a term for fat in the body, usually broken down by the body and used for energy.

lipid profile (LIP-id PRO-file): a blood test that measures levels of total cholesterol, triglycerides, LDL cholesterol, and HDL cholesterol. A lipid profile is a measure of the risk of developing cardiovascular disease.

lipoatrophy (LIPE-oh-A-truh-fee): loss of fat under the skin resulting in small dents; may be caused by repeated injections of insulin in the same spot.

lipodystrophy (LIPE-oh-DIHS-truh-fee): a defect in the breaking down or building up of fat below the surface of the skin, resulting in lumps or small dents in the skin surface; may be caused by repeated injections of insulin in the same spot. *Ex.*: lipohypertrophy, lipoatrophy.

lipohypertrophy (LIPE-oh-hy-PER-truh-fee): buildup of fat below the surface of the skin, causing lumps; may be caused by repeated injections of insulin in the same spot. SYN.: hypertrophy.

lipolysis (LIPE-ah-lih-sis): the breakdown of fat stored in fat cells; this process also releases ketones into the bloodstream.

lipoprotein (lipe-OH-pro-teen): a protein that travels through the bloodstream with the purpose of delivering lipids to cells.

lispro insulin (LYZ-proh IN-suh-lin): a rapid-acting insulin. On average, lispro insulin starts to lower blood glucose levels within 5 minutes after injection and has its strongest effect 30 minutes to 1 hour after injection but keeps working for 3 hours after injection.

liver (LIH-ver): an organ that changes food into energy, removes alcohol and poisons from the blood, stores glycogen, and makes bile, a substance that breaks down fats and helps rid the body of wastes.

K–O

logbook (lawg-book): a book in which readings are kept; for people with diabetes, it can contain blood glucose levels, blood pressure, eating data, and physical activity data.

long-acting insulin (long-ackt-ing IN-suh-lin): a basal insulin that starts to lower blood glucose levels within 4–6 hours after injection and has its strongest effect 10–18 hours after injection. *Ex.*: detemir insulin, glargine insulin.

low-calorie sweetener (LO-CAL-or-ee sweet-en-er): a product used to sweeten foods in place of sugar; does not contain many calories per serving and does not raise blood glucose levels. *Ex.*: saccharin, acesulfame-K, aspartame (NutraSweet), and sucralose (Splenda).

low-density lipoprotein cholesterol (LO-den-SIH-tee LIPE-oh-PRO-teen kuh-LESS-tuh-rawl): a fat that travels in the bloodstream; takes cholesterol around the body to where it is needed for cell repair and also deposits it on the inside of artery walls, sometimes leading to atherosclerosis; often called "bad" or "unhealthy" cholesterol. ABBREV.: LDL cholesterol.

lymphocyte (LIM-foh-syte): a type of white blood cell involved in the human body's immune system that plays an important and integral part in defending the body from illness and disease; there are two broad categories of lymphocytes, namely T cells (T lymphocytes) and B cells (B lymphocytes).

M

macroalbuminuria (MACK-ro-al-BYOO-min-your-EE-ah): a condition characterized by large amounts of albumin in the urine; a sign of future end-stage renal failure.

macrosomia (mack-roh-SOH-mee-ah): abnormally large; in diabetes, refers to abnormally large babies that may be born to women with diabetes.

macrovascular disease (mack-roh-VASK-yoo-ler dih-zeez): disease of the large blood vessels, such as those found in the heart. Lipids and blood clots build up in the large blood vessels and can cause atherosclerosis, coronary heart disease, stroke, and peripheral vascular disease.

K–O

macula (MACK-yoo-la): the part of the retina in the eye used for reading and seeing fine detail.

macular edema (MACK-yoo-lur eh-DEE-mah): swelling of the macula.

managed care (MAN-edged kair): a system of health care that controls costs by placing limits on doctors' fees and by restricting the patient's choice of physicians.

managed-care organization (MAN-edged kair organ-ih-zay-shun): any type of organization that provides managed care to its members, such as an exclusive provider organization, health maintenance organization, or preferred provider organization.

mannitol (MAN-eh-tall): a sugar alcohol that, when taken in excess, has a laxative effect (causes diarrhea); may be used to treat increased pressure in the brain

maturity-onset diabetes of the young (MAH-chur-ih-tee-on-set DY-uh-beet-eez of the yung): a rare form of hereditary diabetes that shares the characteristics of type 2 diabetes and generally develops in young adults. Of the six forms identified, each is caused by a defect in a single gene that impairs insulin secretion; often misdiagnosed as type 1 diabetes in younger patients and as type 2 diabetes in older patients. ABBREV.: MODY.

meal plan (MEEL plan): a guide to healthy eating for people with diabetes that tells the patient what to eat, how much to eat, and when to eat; usually developed with the help of a dietitian.

medical history (med-ih-cull his-tor-ee): a list of a person's previous illnesses, current conditions, symptoms, medications, and health risk factors.

medical nutrition therapy (med-ih-cull NOO-trih-shun thair-uh-pee): the broad-based approach to adding healthy eating to a person's lifestyle in order to improve health outcomes; usually includes promoting the development of a meal plan, education in making healthy food choices, and encouraging more physical activity. This is an important part of the process of preventing diabetes, managing existing dia-

K–O

betes, and preventing the rate of development of diabetes complications. ABBREV.: MNT.

Medicaid (med-ih-CAYD): a federal and state health care insurance assistance program that is provided to people with very low income or who are disabled, senior citizens, or children. The income level at which people can join this program is individually determined by each state.

Medicare (med-ih-KAIR): a federal health care insurance program for people 65 years of age or older and for some people with disabilities who cannot work. There are two main parts of Medicare, Parts A and B. Part A helps pay for medical care provided in hospitals, skilled nursing facilities, hospices, and nursing homes. Part B helps pay for health providers' services, ambulance services, diagnostic tests, outpatient hospital services, outpatient physical therapy, speech pathology services, and medical equipment and supplies. In 2005, Part B was updated to include many diabetes-related services, including diabetes screening tests, diabetes self-management education, medical nutrition therapy, and diabetes supplies, so

Medicare Part B is essential for people with diabetes who qualify for Medicare coverage. Medicare Part D is the voluntary prescription drug insurance program.

Medigap (med-ih-GAP): an additional health care insurance plan that is sold by private insurance companies to pay for some of the costs for which Medicare does not provide coverage (thus, it pays for the "gaps" in Medicare coverage). Plans vary from one insurance company to another, so it is necessary to carefully evaluate the benefits of individual Medigap plans.

meglitinide (meh-GLIH-tin-ide): a class of oral medicine for type 2 diabetes that lowers blood glucose levels by helping the pancreas make more insulin after meals. G.N.: repaglinide.

metabolic syndrome (MET-ah-BALL-ick sin-drohm): a collection of various risk factors that tend to group together in individuals (including obesity, insulin resistance, diabetes, hypertension, and dyslipidemia) and can lead to heart disease. This is not necessarily a disease that is diagnosed, but instead is a tool for esti-

K–O

mating the risk of the development of heart disease. The metabolic syndrome has been the subject of debate among scientists with regard to its usefulness as a diagnosable clinical entity and its diagnosis criteria.

metabolism (MET-ab-ohl-ism): the umbrella term for the way cells chemically change food so that it can be used to store or burn energy and make the proteins, fats, and sugars needed by the body.

metformin (met-FOR-min): an oral medicine belonging to the biguanide class of medications used to treat type 2 diabetes. B.N.: Glucophage, Glucophage XR.

microalbuminuria (MY-kro-al-BYOO-min-your-EE-ah): a condition characterized by small amounts of albumin in the urine; an early sign of nephropathy; usually managed by improving blood glucose control, reducing blood pressure and use of specific antihypertensive medications, and modifying diet.

microaneurysm (MY-kro-AN-yeh-rizm): a small swelling that forms on the side of tiny blood vessels; may break and allow blood to leak into nearby tissue. People with diabetes may have microaneurysms in the retina of the eye.

microvascular disease (MY-kro-VASK-yoo-ler dih-zeez): disease of the smallest blood vessels, such as those found in the eyes, nerves, and kidneys. The walls of the vessels become abnormally thick but weak, and then they bleed, leak protein, and slow the flow of blood to the cells.

miglitol (MIG-lih-tall): an oral medicine used to treat type 2 diabetes that belongs to the class of medicines called alpha-glucosidase inhibitors. B.N.: Glyset.

milligrams per deciliter (MILL-ih-grams per DESS-ih-lee-tur): a unit of measure that shows the concentration of a substance in a specific amount of fluid. In the U.S., used to report blood glucose levels; other countries use millimoles per liter. To convert milligrams per deciliter to millimoles per liter, multiply mmol/l by 18. *Ex.*: 10 mmol/l × 18 = 180 mg/dl. ABBREV.: mg/dl.

millimoles per liter (MILL-ih-mohls per LEE-tur): a unit of measure that shows the concentration of a substance in a specific amount of fluid. For most of the world (except for the U.S.) used to report blood glucose levels. To convert to millimoles per liter to milligrams per deciliter, divide mg/dl by 18. *Ex.*: 180 mg/dl ÷ 18 = 10 mmol/l. ABBREV.: mmol/l.

mixed dose (MIX-d dohs): a combination of two types of insulin in one injection. Typically, a rapid- or short-acting insulin is combined with a longer-acting insulin (such as NPH insulin) to provide both short-term and long-term management of blood glucose levels.

molecule (MAH-leh-kyool): smallest unit of a chemical compound that can exist by itself and retain all of its chemical properties; composed of two or more atoms.

monofilament (MAHN-oh-fill-uh-ment): a short piece of nylon, such as a hairbrush bristle, mounted on a wand that is used to check the sensitivity of the nerves in the foot; a physician touches the filament to the bottom of the foot and the patient says whether he or she can feel the filament touching the foot.

mononeuropathy (MAH-noh-ne-ROP-uh-thee): neuropathy affecting a single nerve.

monounsaturated fat (MAH-no-un-SATCH-ur-AY-ted fat): a type of "healthy" dietary fat that is found in large amounts in foods from plants, particularly olive and canola oil, and including avocados, nuts, and peanut butter; usually in liquid form when at room temperature.

morbid obesity (MORE-bid OH-bees-ity): severe obesity in which a person has a BMI over 40 kg/m^2; usually equivalent to being 100 pounds over ideal body weight.

morbidity (MORE-bid-it-ee): **1.** the state of being ill or diseased; any departure from overall health. **2.** the incidence of disease or sickness within a certain population.

mortality (MORE-tal-ih-tee): a measure of the rate of death from a particular disease within a given population.

myocardial infarction (my-oh-KAR-dee-ul in-FARK-shun): an interruption in the blood supply to the heart because of narrowed or blocked blood vessels, causing muscle damage and possibly death. SYN.: heart attack.

N

nateglinide (neh-TEH-glin-ide): an oral medicine used to treat type 2 diabetes that belongs to the class of medicines called D-phenylalanine derivatives. B.N.: Starlix.

necrobiosis lipoidica diabeticorum (NEK-roh-by-OH-sis lih-POY-dik-ah DY-uh-bet-ih-KOR-um): a skin condition usually on the lower part of the legs that develops in people with diabetes. Lesions can be small or extend over a large area. They are usually raised, yellow, and waxy in appearance and often have a purple border.

necrosis (NECK-ro-sis): the death of cells or tissues of the body as a result of injury, infection, inflammation, or disease; often involves a small area of the body.

K–O

neovascularization (NEE-oh-VASK-yoo-ler-ih-ZAY-shun): the growth of new, small blood vessels. In the retina, this may lead to loss of vision or blindness.

nephrologist (neh-FRAH-luh-jist): a doctor who treats people who have kidney problems.

nephropathy (neh-FROP-uh-thee): disease of the kidneys. Hyperglycemia and hypertension can damage the glomerulus of the kidney. When the kidneys are damaged, they can no longer remove waste and extra fluids from the bloodstream and protein leaks into the urine.

nerve conduction study (nerv kon-duck-shun stuh-dee): a test used to measure for nerve damage; used to diagnose neuropathy. ABBREV.: NCS.

neurogenic bladder (nyur-eh-jeen-ick bla-dur): a state in which the bladder (the organ that contains urine) works improperly due to nerve damage caused by diabetes, stroke, injury, or other conditions; people with this condition may experience urine leakage, difficulty urinat-

K–O

ing, damage to the blood vessels in the kidneys, and urinary tract infections.

neurologist (nyur-RAH-luh-jist): a doctor who specializes in problems of the nervous system, such as neuropathy.

neuropathy (ne-ROP-uh-thee): disease of the nervous system; a complication of diabetes. The three major forms in people with diabetes are peripheral neuropathy, autonomic neuropathy, and mononeuropathy. The most common form is peripheral neuropathy, which primarily affects the legs and feet.

nonalcoholic fatty liver disease (non-AL-koh-hol-ic fat-tee liv-er dih-zeez): a condition characterized by the abnormal presence of fat on the liver that is not due to consumption of alcohol; people who have insulin resistance and/or the metabolic syndrome are at higher risk of developing this condition, though some medications can also increase the chances of getting it; can lead to inflammation of the liver and possibly cirrhosis (when healthy liver tissue is replaced with scar tissue, eventually reducing healthy liver function). ABBREV.: NAFLD.

non–insulin-dependent diabetes mellitus (non-IN-suh-lin-DEE-pen-dent DY-uh-beet-eez MEL-ih-tus): OBS.: type 2 diabetes. [*Usage*: so called because of the perception that this particular form of diabetes was only treated with diet, exercise, and oral hypoglycemic agents; with the beginning of insulin use in patients with NIDDM, this term became less useful.] ABBREV.: NIDDM.

noninvasive blood glucose monitoring (NON-in-VAY-siv blud GLOO-kose mon-i-ter-ing): a method of measuring blood glucose levels without drawing a blood sample. Currently, one approved method (the GlucoWatch G2 Biographer, manufactured by Cygnus Inc.) uses small electric currents to draw fluids from the skin.

nonproliferative retinopathy (non-pro-LIF-er-uh-tiv REH-tih-NOP-uh-thee): SYN.: background retinopathy.

nonsteroidal anti-inflammatory drug (non-stair-OYD-uhl an-tee-in-flam-uh-tor-ee drug): a class of medication that relieves pain, fever, and inflammation; in general, these drugs do not

K–O

have a high risk of addiction or cause sleepiness. *Ex.*: ibuprofen, aspirin, acetaminophen. ABBREV.: NSAID.

normoglycemia (NOR-mo-gly-SEEM-ee-uh): SYN.: euglycemia; steady, normal blood glucose levels.

NPH insulin (en-pee-aytch IN-suh-lin): an intermediate-acting insulin; NPH stands for neutral protamine Hagedorn. Protamine is a protein that, when added to insulin, slows down its onset and duration. NPH insulin starts to lower blood glucose within 1–2 hours after injection and has its strongest effect 6–10 hours after injection but keeps working for about 10 hours after injection. SYN.: N insulin.

nurse (nurs): a health care professional trained in nursing, which is the practice of providing care for those who are ill or injured, often through the use of a prescribed care plan (usually developed by a physician). Nurses are typically responsible for administering medication, assessing a patient's health status, keeping records, and preventing infection. In professional care, there are two classifications of professional nurses: registered nurse and licensed practical nurse. [*Usage*: "nurse" is often used as a synonym for "registered nurse."]

nurse practitioner (nurs PRACK-tish-un-er): a registered nurse who has taken advanced training and received a master's degree in nursing; can perform many of the duties of a physician without supervision; may take on additional duties in diagnosis and treatment of patients. ABBREV.: NP.

Nutrition Facts label (noo-TRIH-shun fackts LAY-bul): a standardized label on any food or beverage providing nutritional information that is required on any food distributed in the U.S. and regulated by the U.S. Food and Drug Administration. This label must contain the following information: serving size, servings per container, calories, calories from fat, total fat, saturated fat, trans fat, cholesterol, sodium, total carbohydrate, dietary fiber, sugars, and protein.

nutritionist (noo-TRIH-shuh-nist): a person with training in nutrition; may or may not have specialized training and qualifications (as opposed to a registered dietitian).

K–O

O

obese (OH-bees): an abnormally high, unhealthy body weight; defined as a body mass index of 30 kg/m^2 or higher.

obesity (OH-bees-ih-TEE): the condition in which a person is obese.

obstetrician (ob-steh-TRIH-shun): a doctor who treats pregnant women and delivers babies.

omega-3 fatty acid (OH-meh-guh-three fat-ee ass-id): a polyunsaturated fat that is mainly found in oily, fatty fish, such as wild salmon, herring, tuna, and anchovies; also found in flaxseed oil; has an anti-inflammatory effect and may be beneficial to heart health. Also written as ω-3 fatty acid.

ophthalmologist (AHF-thal-MAH-luh-jist): a medical doctor who diagnoses and treats all eye diseases and eye disorders; can also prescribe glasses and contact lenses.

optician (ahp-TIH-shun): a health care professional who dispenses glasses and lenses and makes and fits contact lenses.

optometrist (ahp-TAH-meh-trist): a primary eye care provider who prescribes glasses and contact lenses; can diagnose and treat certain eye conditions and diseases.

oral glucose tolerance test (OR-ul GLOO-kose tohl-er-ENTS test): a test to diagnose diabetes or impaired glucose tolerance; administered by a health care professional after an overnight fast; often conducted when it is unclear as to whether a diagnosis of type 1 or type 2 diabetes should be made. A blood sample is taken and then the patient drinks a high-glucose beverage. Blood samples are then taken at intervals for 2–3 hours. ABBREV.: OGTT.

oral hypoglycemic agent (OR-ul HI-po-gly-SEE-mik AY-jent): medicine taken by mouth to keep blood glucose as close to normal as possible; generally prescribed to treat type 2 diabetes. Classes of this medication include alpha-glucosidase inhibitors, biguanides, D-phenylalanine derivatives, meglitinides, sulfonylureas, and thiazolidinediones.

K–O

orthotic (OR-thah-tick): a mechanical device, such as a support or brace, that helps weak or ineffective joints or muscles function. SYN.: orthosis.

orthotist (OR-thuh-tist): a specialist skilled in making orthotics.

osteoporosis (OSS-tee-oh-pa-ROW-sis): a condition characterized by decreased bone mass and density, causing the bones to become fragile and increasingly susceptible to fractures; it can arise in men (especially elderly men) and women but is highly prevalent in women who have passed menopause.

otolaryngologist (OH-tow-lair-in-gahl-uh-jist): a doctor who specializes in the treatment of the ears, nose, and throat.

over-the-counter drug (oh-ver-the-cown-ter drug): a medication that can be purchased without a prescription and without visiting a medical professional. *Ex.*: cold remedies, aspirin. ABBREV.: OTC drug.

overweight (OH-ver-wayt): an above-normal body weight, but not obese; defined as a body mass index of 25–29.9 kg/m^2.

K–O

P

pancreas (PAN-kree-us): a comma-shaped gland located just behind the stomach that produces enzymes for digesting food and hormones that regulate the use of fuels in the body, including insulin and glucagon.

pancreas transplantation (PAN-kree-us trans-plan-TAY-shun): a surgical procedure in which a healthy whole or partial pancreas (one that still makes insulin) is taken from a donor and placed into a person with diabetes, usually type 1 diabetes. Sometimes this procedure also includes the transplantation of kidneys at the same time, called simultaneous kidney pancreas transplantation.

pattern management (PAT-ern man-udj-ment): a method of identifying trends (thus, patterns) in changes in blood glucose levels and adjusting the factors that contribute to these trends to achieve blood glucose levels closer to normal levels. This method requires more work on the part of the patient and collaboration with the health care team, but can help prevent the development of complications. A person who follows pattern management studies records of food, medication, physical activity, and blood glucose levels and learns how to identify and correct trends.

pediatric endocrinologist (pee-dee-AT-rik en-doh-krih-NAH-luh-jist): a doctor who treats children who have endocrine gland problems such as diabetes.

pedometer (ped-ah-met-er): a portable device that counts each step a person takes; some are electronic and can measure distances traveled; frequently used to evaluate the amount of physical activity a person has in an average day.

pedorthist (ped-OR-thist): a health care professional who specializes in fitting shoes for people with disabilities or deformities and can make custom shoes or orthotics (e.g., special inserts for shoes).

percutaneous transluminal coronary angioplasty (per-kyoo-tane-ee-us trans-loo-min-ul core-uh-nair-ee an-gee-UH-plast-EE): SYN.: angioplasty. ABBREV.: PTCA.

periodontal disease (PER-ee-oh-DON-tul dih-zeez): disease of the gums.

periodontist (PER-ee-oh-DON-tist): a dentist who specializes in treating people who have gum diseases.

peripheral arterial disease (PER-ih-fer-ul AR-teer-ee-ul dih-zeez): a disease that occurs when blood vessels in the legs are narrowed or blocked by fatty deposits, reducing blood flow to the feet and legs. This condition puts people at increased risk of heart attack and stroke. One out of every three people with diabetes aged 50 years or older is estimated to have this condition. ABBREV.: PAD.

peripheral neuropathy (PER-ih-fer-ul ne-ROP-uh-thee): nerve damage that affects the feet, legs, or hands; causes pain, numbness, or a tingling feeling. SYN.: distal symmetric polyneuropathy.

peripheral vascular disease (PER-ih-fer-ul VAS-kyoo-ler dih-zeez): a disease of the large blood vessels of the arms, legs, and feet; may occur when major blood vessels in these areas are blocked and do not receive enough blood;

P–T

symptoms include aching pains and slow-healing foot sores. ABBREV.: PVD.

peritoneal dialysis (PARE-ih-tone-ee-ul dy-AL-ih-sis): a type of dialysis that involves passing a special fluid through the abdomen. The waste products pass from the blood, through a membrane lining the inside of the abdomen, and into the special fluid that can then be drained from the body. Unlike hemodialysis, this form of dialysis can be done in the home or at work, and some methods do not even require the use of a machine.

pharmaceutical (FAR-mah-soo-tih-cull): a medicinal drug or having to do with drugs. *Ex.*: a pharmaceutical company is a company that manufactures drugs.

pharmacist (FAR-mah-sist): a health care professional who prepares and distributes medicine to people. Pharmacists also give information on medicines.

photocoagulation (FOH-toh-koh-ag-yoo-LAY-shun): a laser surgery treatment for diabetic retinopathy. A strong beam of light (laser) is used to seal off bleeding blood vessels in the eye and to burn away extra blood vessels that should not have grown there.

physical activity (fis-ih-cull ack-tiv-ih-tee): any form of exercise or movement, including walking, running, sports, and regular day-to-day activities, such as yard work, walking the dog, cleaning, and running errands. Adults should try to get at least 30 minutes of moderate physical activity (any activity that requires about as much energy as walking 2 miles in 30 minutes) at least 5 days a week.

physician (FIZZ-ih-shun): a licensed doctor.

physician assistant (FIZZ-ih-shun uh-sis-TENT): a health care professional who is trained and licensed to practice medicine under the guidance of a supervising physician.

pill organizer (pil or-gan-EYE-zer): a small box that has several smaller partitions used to hold different pills; particularly useful for people who take a lot of different oral medications at different times of the day and over different days. The partitions are usually separated into individual days and times of days (e.g., break-fast or morning, lunch or afternoon).

pioglitazone (PIE-oh-GLIT-uh-zone): an oral med-icine used to treat type 2 diabetes that belongs to the class of medicines called thiazolidine-diones. B.N.: Actos.

pituitary gland (pit-ew-ih-tair-ee gland): an endocrine gland at the base of the brain that produces hormones and helps regulate metab-olism, blood pressure, growth, and thyroid gland function.

plaque (plak): hardened deposits that form on the inner walls of blood vessels.

plasma (PLAZ-muh): the yellow liquid part of blood that contains water, proteins, elec-trolytes, sugars (e.g., glucose), lipids, meta-bolic waste products (e.g., urea), amino acids, hormones, and vitamins. SYN.: blood plasma.

podiatrist (puh-DY-uh-trist): a doctor who treats people who have foot problems; also helps people keep their feet healthy by providing regular foot examinations and treatment.

podiatry (puh-DY-uh-tree): the care and treatment of feet.

point system (poynt sis-tem): a meal-planning system that uses points to rate the calorie content of foods. *Ex.*: Weight Watchers.

polycystic ovary syndrome (pah-lee-sis-tick oh-ver-ee sin-drome): a hormonal disorder that affects young women of reproductive age and can cause infertility in some patients; many patients with this disorder also have insulin resistance; some symptoms include infrequent or nonexistent periods, acne, obesity, and excess hair growth. ABBREV.: PCOS.

polydipsia (pah-lee-DIP-see-uh): excessive thirst; may be a sign of diabetes.

polyol (PAH-lee-all): SYN.: sugar alcohol.

polypeptide (pah-lee-PEP-tide): chains of amino acids that consist of up to about 50 amino acids and are created by living systems.

polyphagia (pah-lee-FAY-jee-ah): excessive hunger; may be a sign of diabetes.

P–T

polyunsaturated fat (pah-lee-un-SATCH-ur-AY-ted fat): a type of "healthy" dietary fat that is found in large amounts in foods from plants, particularly vegetable oils, such as those from safflower, sunflower, cottonseed, soybean, and corn; can also be found in margarine; usually in liquid form when at room temperature.

polyuria (pah-lee-YOOR-ee-ah): excessive urination; may be a sign of diabetes.

portion control (por-shun kon-trol): the process of eating sensible serving sizes; essential for achieving weight loss and maintaining a healthy body weight; a key tactic in meal planning.

postprandial (post-PRAN-dee-ul): after a meal. A postprandial blood glucose level is one taken 1–2 hours after eating.

pramlintide (pram-lin-tide): an injectable medication for the treatment of diabetes that is a synthetic form of the hormone amylin. Pramlintide injections taken with meals have been shown to modestly improve A1C levels without causing increased hypoglycemia or weight gain; it even promotes slight weight loss. The primary side

P–T

effect is nausea, which tends to improve over time and as an individual patient determines his or her optimal dose. B.N.: Symlin.

pre-diabetes (pree-DY-uh-beet-eez): a condition in which blood glucose levels are higher than normal but are not high enough for a diagnosis of diabetes. People with pre-diabetes are at increased risk for developing type 2 diabetes and for heart disease and stroke. Also called impaired glucose tolerance and impaired fasting glucose.

preeclampsia (PREE-ih-clamp-see-uh): a serious condition in which pregnant women develop hypertension, begin swelling due to fluid retention, and develop proteinuria; more common in women with diabetes. SYN.: toxemia.

preferred provider organization (PREE-ferd PRO-vi-dur or-gan-ih-zay-shun): a managed-care plan that arranges coverage for specific services through a network of participating providers that is contracted by the insurance company. Under this type of plan, most health care costs are covered when a network physician is visited. ABBREV.: PPO.

P–T

premixed insulin (pree-mix-d IN-suh-lin): a commercially produced combination of two different types of insulin. *Ex.*: 50/50 insulin and 70/30 insulin.

preprandial (pree-PRAN-dee-ul): before a meal.

prevalence (prev-UH-lents): the number of people in a given group or population who are reported to have a disease.

preventive treatment (pre-ven-tive treet-ment): a treatment or therapy that is intended to preserve health and prevent the development of a disease or complications.

progesterone (PRO-jest-uh-rohn): a female hormone that helps prepare the uterus (the womb) to receive and sustain the fertilized egg; during the menstrual cycle in some women, progesterone may cause blood glucose levels to fluctuate.

proinsulin (proh-IN-suh-lin): the substance made in the beta cells and split into several products, one of which is insulin.

proliferative retinopathy (pro-LIH-fur-ah-tiv REH-tih-NOP-uh-thee): a condition in which fragile new blood vessels grow along the retina and in the vitreous humor of the eye, which can cause blood to leak into the clear fluid inside the eye and can also cause the retina to detach; sometimes leads to loss of vision (blindness).

prosthesis (prahs-THEE-sis): a man-made substitute for a missing body part such as an arm or a leg.

prosthetist (prahs-THEH-tist): a person involved in the science and art of prosthetics; one who designs and fits artificial limbs.

protein (PRO-teen): **1.** one of the main nutrients in food. Foods that provide protein include meat, poultry, fish, cheese, milk, dairy products, eggs, and dried beans. **2.** proteins are used by the body to build cell structure, make hormones such as insulin, and for other various functions.

proteinuria (PRO-tee-NOOR-ee-uh): the presence of protein in the urine, indicating that the kidneys are not working properly.

P–T

psychiatrist (SYE-kye-uh-trist): a medical doctor who specializes in the evaluation, diagnosis, and treatment of mental disorders; can prescribe medications.

psychologist (SYE-koll-uh-jist): a specialist who treats people through counseling in an attempt to help overcome emotional or psychological reactions to injury, disease, or other experiences; cannot prescribe medications.

pulse (puhls): **1.** the heart beat felt throbbing through an artery; usually felt in the neck or wrist. **2.** the number of times the heart beats in 1 minute. SYN.: heart rate.

R

random plasma glucose test (ran-DUM PLAZ-muh GLOO-kose test): a test in which blood is drawn at any point in the day, regardless of whether the subject is fasting, to determine blood glucose levels; if blood glucose levels are abnormal, a fasting plasma glucose test will usually be used to diagnose diabetes. SYN.: casual plasma glucose test.

P–T

rapid-acting insulin (ra-pid-ackt-ing IN-suh-lin): a type of insulin that starts to lower blood glucose levels within 5–10 minutes after injection and has its strongest effect 30 minutes to 3 hours after injection, depending on the type used. *Ex.*: aspart insulin, lispro insulin.

rebound hyperglycemia (REE-bownd HY-per-gly-SEE-mee-uh): a swing to high blood glucose levels after hypoglycemia. SYN.: Somogyi effect.

receptor (REE-sep-tur): a molecule on the surface of a cell that binds to a specific substance and causes a change in the way that the cell works.

Recognized Diabetes Education Program (RECK-ug-NIZE-d DY-uh-beet-eez ed-joo-kay-shun PRO-gram): diabetes self-management education programs that meet the American Diabetes Association's National Standards for Diabetes Self-Management Education.

Recommended Dietary Allowance (RECK-oh-mend-ed DY-eh-tarry UH-low-ants): one of the four reference values of the Dietary Reference Intake; the average daily intake level that is sufficient to meet the nutrient requirements of

P–T

nearly all healthy individuals of a particular age and gender. ABBREV.: RDA.

red blood cell (red blud sel): a cell in blood plasma that contains hemoglobin, which allows it to carry oxygen to all parts of the body. SYN.: erythrocyte. ABBREV.: RBC.

registered dietitian (rej-ih-sterd DY-eh-TIH-shun): a dietitian who has had further education and training in order to earn credentials from the Commission on Accreditation for Dietetics Education, an agency of the American Dietetic Association. ABBREV.: RD.

registered nurse (rej-ih-sterd nurs): a nurse who has taken 2 or more years of education and training in providing nursing care and received licensing from a certified school. ABBREV.: RN.

regular insulin (reg-yoo-lur IN-suh-lin): a short-acting insulin that has properties that mimic those of insulin produced by the body. On average, regular insulin starts to lower blood glucose levels within 30 minutes after injection and has its strongest effect 2–5 hours after injection but keeps working for 5–8 hours after injection. SYN.: R insulin.

P-T

renal (REE-nal): having to do with the kidneys.

renal disease (REE-nal dih-zeez): a disease of the kidneys. SYN.: nephropathy.

repaglinide (reh-PAG-lih-nide): an oral medicine used to treat type 2 diabetes that belongs to the class of medicines called meglitinides. B.N.: Prandin.

retina (REH-ti-nuh): the light-sensitive layer of tissue that lines the back of the eye.

retinopathy (REH-tih-NOP-uh-thee): damage to small blood vessels in the eye that can lead to vision problems; different forms include background retinopathy and proliferative retinopathy.

risk factor (risk fack-tor): anything that raises the chances of a person developing a disease.

rosiglitazone (rose-ee-GLIH-tuh-zone): an oral medicine used to treat type 2 diabetes that belongs to the class of medicines called thiazolidinediones. B.N.: Avandia.

P–T

S

saccharin (SAK-ah-rin): an artificial low-calorie sweetener with no calories and no nutritional value.

saturated fat (SATCH-ur-AY-ted fat): a fat found mainly in animal-based foods, such as meat and dairy products, but also in some oils, such as palm oil and coconut oil; can raise LDL cholesterol levels, so it is a fat to be avoided or reduced in the diet; is often a solid fat when at room temperature.

secondary diabetes (sec-und-airy DY-uh-beet-eez): a type of diabetes that develops because of the effects of another disease or because of reactions to certain drugs or chemicals.

sedentary lifestyle (sed-en-TAIR-ee LYFE-stile): a way of life characterized by a lack of physical activity; in general, people in Western civilizations follow a sedentary lifestyle.

self-management (self-man-udj-ment): in diabetes and other chronic diseases, the ongoing process of managing the disease by the patient in collaboration with a health care team; for diabetes, includes meal planning, planned physical activity, blood glucose monitoring, taking diabetes medicines, handling episodes of illness, managing diabetes when traveling, and more.

self-monitoring of blood glucose (self-mon-ih-ter-ing of blud GLOO-kose): the process by which a person with diabetes checks, records, and evaluates his or her own blood glucose levels; an essential component of pattern management and the key to diabetes self-care. ABBREV.: SMBG.

serum (SEER-um): the yellowish liquid part of blood that is obtained from clotted blood; serum is very similar to plasma except that the clotting factors (proteins that make blood clot) have been removed by clot formation. Also called also blood serum.

serving size (ser-ving size): **1.** the size of a portion of food that is eaten in one sitting; in many cases, people eat meals in which the serving size is too large, contributing to over-

P–T

weight and obesity. **2.** a listing on a Nutrition Facts label that identifies how much of a certain food constitutes one serving.

70/30 insulin (sev-en-tee thir-tee IN-suh-lin): premixed insulin that consists of 70% intermediate-acting (NPH) insulin and 30% short-acting (regular) insulin.

sharps container (sharps kon-tayn-er): a container into which used needles and syringes are disposed; often made of hard plastic so that needles cannot poke through.

short-acting insulin (short-ackt-ing IN-suh-lin): a type of insulin that starts to lower blood glucose levels within 30 minutes after injection and has its strongest effect 2–5 hours after injection. *Ex.*: regular insulin.

side effect (side eh-feckt): an unintended action of a drug. SYN.: adverse effect.

simultaneous kidney pancreas transplantation (SY-mull-TANE-ee-us KID-nee PAN-kree-us trans-plan-TAY-shun): a surgical procedure in which a healthy whole or partial pancreas (one

P–T

that still makes insulin) and functioning kidneys are taken from a donor and placed into a person with type 1 diabetes and end-stage renal disease. ABBREV.: SKP transplant.

sitagliptin (sit-uh-glip-tin): an oral hypoglycemic agent used to treat type 2 diabetes and belonging to the class of medications called dipeptidyl peptidase-IV inhibitors. B.N.: Januvia.

sodium (SOH-dee-um): a mineral and dietary nutrient that helps maintain the balance of water in the cells and keeps nerves functioning; most dietary sodium comes in the form of table salt or salt added to processed foods; can contribute to high blood pressure.

soluble fiber (soll-you-buhl FY-bur): dietary fiber found in foods such as oats, barley, fruits, and vegetables; can help improve serum lipid levels.

Somogyi effect (suh-MOH-jee eh-feckt): when blood glucose levels swing high after a hypoglycemic episode; may follow an untreated hypoglycemic episode during the night and is caused by the release of counterregulatory hormones. SYN.: rebound hyperglycemia.

sorbitol (SORE-bih-tall): **1.** a sugar alcohol (sweetener) with 2.6 calories per gram. **2.** a substance produced by the body in people with diabetes that can cause damage to the eyes and nerves.

split mixed dose (split mix-d dohs): the division of a prescribed daily dose of insulin into two or more injections given over the course of the day.

starch (starch): one of the three main types of carbohydrate; dietary sources include beans, lentils, peas, grains, breads, and starchy vegetables (such as peas, potatoes, and corn). SYN.: complex carbohydrate.

strength training (strayn-kth TRAY-ning): activities specifically designed to build muscle and increase strength.

stress hormone (stress HORE-mown): SYN.: counterregulatory hormone.

stroke (strohk): a serious condition caused by damage to blood vessels in the brain, thereby stopping the flow of blood and oxygen to the

P–T

brain, possibly causing brain cells to die; may cause loss of ability to speak or to move parts of the body; risk factors include diabetes, hypertension, high cholesterol (dyslipidemia), and smoking. SYN.: cerebrovascular accident (CVA).

subclinical diabetes (sub-clin-ih-cul DY-uh-beet-eez): OBS.; SYN.: impaired glucose tolerance.

subcutaneous (sub-kyoo-TAY-nee-us in-JEK-shun): when a fluid is put into the tissue under the skin. ABBREV.: SC.

sucralose (soo-cruh-LOHS): an artificial low-calorie sweetener with very few calories and no nutritional value. B.N.: Splenda.

sucrose (soo-KROHS): a simple sugar that the body breaks down into glucose and fructose; also known as table sugar or white sugar, it is found naturally in sugar cane and in beets.

sugar (shoo-ger): **1.** one of the three main types of carbohydrate; characterized by a sweet taste; includes glucose, fructose, lactose, galactose, and sucrose. **2.** sometimes used to refer to blood glucose (e.g., blood sugar).

P–T

sugar alcohol (shoo-ger al-ko-hol): a sweetener that produces a smaller rise in blood glucose than other carbohydrates; contains about 2 calories per gram; includes erythritol, isomalt, lactitol, maltitol, mannitol, sorbitol, and xylitol. Also known as polyol.

sugar diabetes (shoo-ger DY-uh-beet-eez): OBS.; SYN.: diabetes mellitus.

sugar substitute (shoo-ger sub-stih-toot): a substance used to sweeten foods; used in place of sugar. Some sugar substitutes have calories and will affect blood glucose levels, such as fructose and sugar alcohols (e.g., sorbitol and mannitol). Others have very few calories and will not affect blood glucose levels, such as the low-calorie sweeteners: saccharin, acesulfame-K, aspartame (NutraSweet), and sucralose (Splenda).

sulfonylurea (sul-fah-nil-yoor-EE-uh): a class of oral medication for type 2 diabetes that lowers blood glucose levels by helping the beta cells make more insulin. The most common side effect of this class of drug is hypoglycemia. G.N.: acetohexamide, chlorpropamide, glimepiride, glipizide, glyburide, tolazamide, tolbutamide.

Syndrome X (sin-drohm ecks): OBS.; SYN.: metabolic syndrome.

syringe (suh-RINJ): a device used to inject medications or other liquids into body tissues. The syringe for insulin has a hollow plastic tube with a plunger inside and a needle on the end.

sweetener (sweet-en-er): SYN.: low-calorie sweetener.

T

tachycardia (TACK-ee-car-DEE-uh): a rapid heart beat (generally over 100 beats per minute) that normally arises from stress or exercise, but can also be a sign of heart problems.

T cell (TEE sel): a type of lymphocyte that attacks virus-infected cells, foreign cells, and cancer cells; plays a critical role in the function of the human immune system. SYN.: T lymphocyte.

P–T

team management (TEEM man-udj-ment): a diabetes treatment approach in which medical care is provided by a health care team, usually consisting of a doctor, a dietitian, a nurse, a diabetes educator, and others. The team acts as advisers to the person with diabetes.

telehealth (TELL-eh-helth): SYN.: telemedicine. [*Usage*: this term is generally a synonym for telemedicine. However, some prefer to define telehealth as the broad system of applying medical care through the use of telecommunications technologies, including administrative, prognostic, and preventive services, whereas, in contrast, telemedicine is concerned only with treatment.]

telemedicine (TELL-eh-med-ih-sin): the use of telecommunications technologies (such as telephones, video conferencing, and the Internet) to deliver medical care from a distance, particularly medical diagnoses, patient care, and consultations; especially useful in rural areas, where access to certain types of advanced care may not be readily available or nearby. SYN.: telehealth (see *Usage* note).

testosterone (test-ah-ster-own): the primary male hormone released by both the adrenal gland and the testicles; promotes the development of male characteristics, but is also present in smaller quantities in women.

thiazide diuretic (THIE-uh-ZYDE DY-ur-eh-tick): a class of antihypertensive drug.

thiazolidinedione (THIGH-uh-ZOH-lih-deen-DYE-own): a class of oral medicine for type 2 diabetes that helps insulin take glucose from the blood into the cells for energy by making cells more sensitive to insulin. G.N.: pioglitazone, rosiglitazone.

thyroid gland (THI-royd gland): an endocrine gland in the neck that regulates growth and metabolism.

tolazamide (tohl-AH-zah-mide): an oral medicine used to treat type 2 diabetes that belongs to the class of medicines called sulfonylureas. B.N.: Tolinase.

P–T

tolbutamide (tohl-BYOO-tah-mide): an oral medicine used to treat type 2 diabetes that belongs to the class of medicines called sulfonylureas. B.N.: Orinase.

Tolerable Upper Intake Level (TOL-er-uh-bul upper in-tayke lev-el): one of the four reference values of the Dietary Reference Intake; the highest level of daily intake of a nutrient that will likely not increase the risk of developing an adverse health effect. If intake increases beyond the Tolerable Upper Intake Level, then the risk of adverse effects increases. ABBREV.: UL.

trans fatty acid (trans fat-ee ass-id): a fat that is produced when liquid fat (oil) is turned into solid fat through a chemical process called hydrogenation; found in foods such as margarine, shortening, and baked foods (e.g., cookies, crackers, muffins, and cereals); eating a large amount of trans fatty acids can raise LDL cholesterol, thus increasing the risk of heart disease. SYN.: trans fat.

P–T

transient ischemic attack (trans-ee-ent is-KEE-mick uh-tack): a temporary blockage or shortage in the blood supply to the brain that can result in temporary changes in vision, balance, and speech; these symptoms generally go away within 24 hours; often called a mini-stroke, but can be an important sign of a future, permanent stroke. ABBREV.: TIA.

triglyceride (try-GLISS-er-ide): the storage form of fat in the body.

type 1 diabetes (tipe wan DY-uh-beet-eez): a less common form of diabetes mellitus, once called juvenile diabetes; characterized by high blood glucose levels caused by a total lack of insulin; occurs when the body's immune system attacks the insulin-producing beta cells in the pancreas and destroys them. The pancreas then produces little or no insulin. Type 1 diabetes develops most often in young people but can appear in adults. It is primarily treated with insulin therapy, meal planning, exercise, and self-monitoring of blood glucose. ABBREV.: T1DM, T1D.

P–T

type 2 diabetes (tipe too DY-uh-beet-eez): the most common form of diabetes mellitus; characterized by high blood glucose levels caused by either a lack of insulin or the body's inability to properly use insulin (insulin resistance) or both. Type 2 diabetes develops most often in middle-aged and older adults but can appear in young people; most people who develop this disease tend to be overweight or obese. It is primarily treated with meal planning, exercise, oral hypoglycemic agents, self-monitoring of blood glucose, and insulin therapy. ABBREV.: T2DM, T2D.

U

ulcer (UL-sur): a deep, open sore or break in the skin.

Ultralente insulin (UL-truh-LEN-tay IN-suh-lin): a long-acting insulin. On average, it starts to lower blood glucose levels within 4–6 hours after injection and has its strongest effect 10–18 hours after injection but keeps working for 24–28 hours after injection. As of 2005, this insulin is no longer manufactured.

U–Z

unit of insulin (YOO-nit of IN-suh-lin): the basic measure of the biological effects of a standardized amount of insulin; equal to 45.5 micrograms of pure, crystallized insulin; sometimes presented as 1 international unit, 1 IU, or 1 UI. In practice, however, one only needs to know how many units of insulin need to be taken for a specific purpose, not what amount of insulin to which the unit is equivalent. *Ex.*: U-100 insulin means that there are 100 units of insulin per milliliter of solution.

United Kingdom Prospective Diabetes Study (YOO-nie-ted KING-dum PRO-speck-tive DY-uh-beet-eez stuh-DEE): a British study conducted from 1977 to 1997 in people with type 2 diabetes; showed that if people lowered blood glucose levels, they also lowered the risk of developing retinopathy and nephropathy. In addition, those with type 2 diabetes and hypertension who lowered blood pressure also reduced their risk of stroke, retinopathy, and death from long-term complications. ABBREV.: UKPDS.

urea (yoo-REE-uh): a waste product found in the blood that results from the normal breakdown

U–Z

of protein in the liver; normally removed from the blood by the kidneys and then excreted in the urine.

uremia (yoo-REE-mee-ah): an illness associated with the buildup of urea in the blood because the kidneys are not working effectively; a sign of kidney failure; symptoms may include nausea, vomiting, loss of appetite, weakness, and confusion.

urine (yoo-RIN): the liquid waste product filtered from the blood by the kidneys, stored in the bladder, and expelled from the body by urination.

urine testing (yoo-RIN test-ing): a test of a urine sample used to diagnose diseases of the urinary system and other body systems; may also be checked for signs of bleeding; for people with diabetes, used to check for the presence of ketones, albumin, and/or glucose (this is done infrequently due to its lack of accuracy). Some tests use a single urine sample, whereas others may require a 24-hour collection. SYN.: urinalysis.

U–Z

urologist (yoo-RAH-luh-jist): a doctor who treats people who have urinary tract problems; also cares for men who have problems with their genital organs, such as erectile dysfunction.

V

vaccination (vax-ih-nay-shun): a process of immunization that is intended to confer immunity to a specific disease; conducted by administering a weakened form of a disease in order to provoke an immune response that will provide immunity to a more serious form of the disease. This procedure works because the human immune system can develop the ability to quickly respond to a disease after it has been exposed to it before.

vardenafil (VAR-den-uh-fill): a drug used to treat erectile dysfunction. B.N.: Levitra.

vascular (VAS-kyoo-ler): of or relating to the body's blood vessels.

vein (vayn): a blood vessel that carries blood to the heart.

U–Z

very-low-calorie diet (VAR-ee-LO-CAL-or-ee DY-et): a short-term weight-loss diet that provides fewer than 1,000 calories per day; usually prescribed for morbidly obese patients who must lose weight quickly in order to survive, therefore it is administered under the supervision of a health care provider; sometimes it is given in the form of a 800-calorie liquid formulas to replace daily meals, but it can also simply be a diet with a very low calorie content. ABBREV.: VLCD.

very-low-density lipoprotein cholesterol (VAR-ee-LO-den-SIH-tee LIPE-oh-PRO-teen kuh-LESS-tuh-rawl): a type of cholesterol that transports triglycerides in the blood; some of this is converted to LDL cholesterol; high levels may be related to cardiovascular disease. ABBREV.: VLDL cholesterol.

vildagliptin (vihl-duh-glip-tin): an oral hypoglycemic agent used to treat type 2 diabetes that belongs to the dipeptidyl peptidase-IV inhibitor class of medications. B.N.: Galvus.

virus (VY-rus): a tiny, parasitic organism that multiplies within cells and causes disease.

U–Z

vitamin (VY-tah-min): an organic substance that living organisms require in very small quantities for good health; normally, the organism cannot create the vitamins itself and instead must obtain it from the diet, either from foods or from dietary supplements (e.g., pills).

vitrectomy (vih-TREK-tuh-mee): a surgical procedure in which the cloudy vitreous humor is removed from the eye and replaced with a salt solution in order to restore sight.

vitreous humor (VIH-tree-us HEW-mer): the clear gel that lies behind the lens of the eye and in front of the retina.

void (voyd): to urinate; to empty the bladder.

W

waist circumference (wayst SIR-cum-fer-ents): measurement of the size of the waist; used to estimate the risks of a person developing obesity-related health problems. Women with a waist measurement of more than 35 inches or men with a waist measurement of more than

40 inches have a higher risk of developing diabetes, hypertension, and heart disease.

white blood cell (white blud sel): a type of cell in the immune system that helps the body fight infection and disease; there are many types, including lymphocytes and macrophages. ABBREV.: WBC.

whole grain (hole grayn): a food in which the whole kernels of a grain (e.g., barley, corn, oats, wheat, rye) are used; believed to provide greater health benefits because it contains a lot of dietary fiber, antioxidants, minerals, and vitamins. Common whole-grain products include oatmeal, popcorn, brown rice, whole-wheat flour, and whole-wheat bread.

wound care (woond kair): steps taken to ensure that a wound (e.g., foot ulcer) heals correctly. People with diabetes need to take special precautions so wounds do not become infected.

U–Z

X

xylitol (ZY-lih-tall): a carbohydrate-based sugar alcohol that is found in plants and used as a sugar substitute; provides calories; found in some mints and chewing gum.

List of
Common Acronyms
and Abbreviations

ACE: angiotensin-converting enzyme
AER: albumin excretion rate
AI: Adequate Intake
AGE: advanced glycosylation end product
ARB: angiotensin receptor blocker
BG: blood glucose
BMI: body mass index
BP: blood pressure
BUN: blood urea nitrogen
CABG: coronary artery bypass graft
CAD: coronary artery disease
CAM: complementary and alternative
  medicine

CBGM: capillary blood glucose monitoring

CDE: certified diabetes educator

CFRD: cystic fibrosis–related diabetes

CGMS: continuous glucose monitoring system

CHD: coronary heart disease

CHF: congestive heart failure

CHO: carbohydrate

COBRA: Consolidated Omnibus Budget Reconciliation Act

COPD: chronic obstructive pulmonary disease

CRP: C-reactive protein

CSII: continuous subcutaneous insulin infusion

CVA: cerebrovascular accident (see stroke)

CVD: cardiovascular disease

DASH: Dietary Approaches to Stop Hypertension study

DCCT: Diabetes Control and Complications Trial

DKA: diabetic ketoacidosis

DME company: Durable Medical Equipment company

DN: diabetic neuropathy

DNA: deoxyribonucleic acid

DPP: Diabetes Prevention Program

DPP-IV or **-4:** dipeptidyl peptidase-IV

DRI: Dietary Reference Intake

EAR: Estimated Average Requirement

ED: erectile dysfunction

EPO: exclusive provider organization

ESRD: end-stage renal disease

FPG: fasting plasma glucose test

GAD antibody: glutamic acid decarboxylase antibody

GDM: gestational diabetes mellitus

GHb: glycosylated hemoglobin

GIP: gastric inhibitory polypeptide or glucose-dependent insulinotropic peptide

GLP-1: glucagon-like peptide-1

GTT: glucose tolerance test

HbA$_{1c}$: glycosylated hemoglobin

HDL cholesterol: high-density lipoprotein cholesterol

HHS: hyperosmolar hyperglycemic syndrome

HHNS: hyperosmolar hyperglycemic nonketotic syndrome

HIPAA: Health Insurance Portability and Accountability Act of 1996

HLA: human leukocyte antigen

HMO: health maintenance organization

HTN: hypertension

IAA: insulin autoantibody

ICA: islet cell autoantibody

IDDM: insulin-dependent diabetes mellitus

IDEA: Individuals with Disabilities in Education Act

IEP: Individualized Education Program

IFG: impaired fasting glucose

IGT: impaired glucose tolerance

IV: intravenous

LADA: latent autoimmune diabetes in adults

LDL cholesterol: low-density lipoprotein cholesterol

LJM: limited joint mobility

LPN: licensed practical nurse

LVN: licensed vocational nurse

mg/dl: milligrams per deciliter

mmol/l: millimoles per liter

MNT: medical nutrition therapy

MODY: maturity-onset diabetes of the young

NAFLD: nonalcoholic fatty liver disease

NCS: nerve conduction study

NIDDM: non–insulin-dependent diabetes mellitus

NP: nurse practitioner

NPH: neutral protamine Hagedorn

NSAID: nonsteroidal anti-inflammatory drug

OGTT: oral glucose tolerance test

OTC drug: over-the-counter drug

PAD: peripheral arterial disease

PCOS: polycystic ovary syndrome

PPO: preferred provider organization

PTCA: percutaneous transluminal coronary angioplasty

PVD: peripheral vascular disease

RBC: red blood cell

RD: registered dietitian

RDA: Recommended Dietary Allowance

RN: registered nurse

SC: subcutaneous

SKP transplant: simultaneous kidney pancreas transplantation

SMBG: self-monitoring of blood glucose

T1D or **T1DM**: type 1 diabetes

T2D or **T2DM**: type 2 diabetes

TIA: transient ischemic attack

U: unit (of insulin)

UKPDS: United Kingdom Prospective Diabetes Study

UL: Tolerable Upper Intake Level

VLCD: very-low-calorie diet

VLDL cholesterol: very-low-density lipoprotein cholesterol

WBC: white blood cell

Other Titles Available from the American Diabetes Association

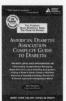

American Diabetes Association Complete Guide to Diabetes, 4th Edition
by the American Diabetes Association
Have all the tips and information on diabetes that you need close at hand. The world's largest collection of diabetes self-care tips, techniques, and tricks for solving diabetes-related problems is back in its fourth edition, and it's bigger and better than ever before. Order no. 4809-04; Price $29.95

Diabetes Fit Food
by Ellen Haas
Put tasteless, boring recipes in the past with this new diabetes cookbook from healthy-eating expert Ellen Haas. She has compiled amazing, healthy recipes from some of America's best celebrity chefs, including Todd English, Alice Waters, and others. Finally, you can make sensible, healthy eating taste like it comes from a five-star restaurant. Order no. 4661-01; Price $16.95

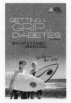

Getting a Grip on Diabetes, 2nd Edition
by Spike Nasmyth Loy and Bo Nasmyth Loy
For children learning to navigate the world of type 1 diabetes comes this revised guide from the people who have firsthand experience. Spike and Bo, who both have had type 1 diabetes since they were children, teach kids of all ages everything they need to know about managing diabetes, including recognizing hypoglycemia, going to college, and traveling safely. Order no. 4909-02; Price $14.95

American Diabetes Association Blood Glucose Log Book
by the American Diabetes Association
Get your blood glucose numbers under control with this handy logbook from the American Diabetes Association. One booklet includes 3 months' worth of blood glucose record sheets, a food diary, charts for your diabetes numbers, and handy guidelines for great diabetes management. Single (3 months): Order no. 5019-01; Price $1.95. Four Pack (1 year): Order no. 5025-01; Price $4.95.

Dr. Buynak's 1-2-3 Diabetes Diet
by Robert J. Buynak and Gregory L. Guthrie
Forget fad diets. Using three simple and sensible steps, this book shows you how to achieve success in healthy eating, calorie counting, exercising, eating out healthfully, resisting temptations, and keeping a positive attitude. It's not always easy, but Dr. Buynak will show you that losing weight is as straightforward as 1-2-3. Order no. 4881-01; Price $14.95

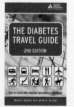

The Diabetes Travel Guide, 2nd Edition
by Davida F. Kruger
Newly revised and updated to include the latest travel guidelines, this thorough, pocket-size guide covers all of the essentials—from planning and packing, to rules on insulin, directives for diabetes pills, health insurance for overseas travel, and what to do if you get sick. Also includes a diabetes phrase book with helpful translations for 8 different languages. Order no. 4836-02; Price $14.95

About the
American Diabetes Association

The American Diabetes Association is the nation's leading voluntary health organization supporting diabetes research, information, and advocacy. Its mission is to prevent and cure diabetes and to improve the lives of all people affected by diabetes. The American Diabetes Association is the leading publisher of comprehensive diabetes information. Its huge library of practical and authoritative books for people with diabetes covers every aspect of self-care—cooking and nutrition, fitness, weight control, medications, complications, emotional issues, and general self-care.

To order American Diabetes Association books: Call 1-800-232-6733 or log on to http://store.diabetes.org

To join the American Diabetes Association: Call 1-800-806-7801 or log on to www.diabetes.org/membership

For more information about diabetes or ADA programs and services: Call 1-800-342-2383. E-mail: AskADA@diabetes.org or log on to www.diabetes.org

To locate an ADA/NCQA Recognized Provider of quality diabetes care in your area: www.ncqa.org/dprp

To find an ADA Recognized Education Program in your area: Call 1-800-342-2383. www.diabetes.org/for-health-professionals-and-scientists/recognition/edrecognition.jsp

To join the fight to increase funding for diabetes research, end discrimination, and improve insurance coverage: Call 1-800-342-2383. www.diabetes.org/advocacy-and-legalresources/advocacy.jsp

To find out how you can get involved with the programs in your community: Call 1-800-342-2383. See below for program Web addresses.

    American Diabetes Month: educational activities aimed at those diagnosed with diabetes—month of November. www.diabetes.org/communityprograms-and-localevents/americandiabetesmonth.jsp

    American Diabetes Alert: annual public awareness campaign to find the undiagnosed—held the fourth Tuesday in March. www.diabetes.org/communityprograms-and-localevents/americandiabetesalert.jsp

    American Diabetes Association Latino Initiative: diabetes awareness program targeted to the Latino community.

www.diabetes.org/communityprograms-and-localevents/latinos.jsp

African American Program: diabetes awareness program targeted to the African American community. www.diabetes.org/communityprograms-and-localevents/africanamericans.jsp

Awakening the Spirit: Pathways to Diabetes Prevention & Control: diabetes awareness program for the Native American community. www.diabetes.org/communityprograms-and-localevents/nativeamericans.jsp

To find out about an important research project regarding type 2 diabetes: www.diabetes.org/diabetes-research/research-home.jsp

To obtain information on making a planned gift or charitable bequest: Call 1-888-700-7029. www.wpg.cc/stl/CDA/homepage/1,1006,509,00.html

To make a donation or memorial contribution: Call 1-800-342-2383. www.diabetes.org/support-the-cause/make-a-donation.jsp